The Chronic Mental Patient/II

Edited by

W. Walter Menninger, M.D.
*Executive Vice President and Chief of Staff,
The Menninger Foundation*

Gerald T. Hannah, Ph.D.
*Commissioner,
Kansas State Office of Mental Health and
Retardation Services,
Topeka*

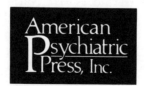

1400 K Street, N.W.
Washington, DC 20005

Library of Congress Cataloging-in-Publication Data

The Chronic mental patient/II.

Based on papers presented at the Second National Conference on the Chronic Mental Patient, held in Kansas City, Mo., August 12–14, 1984.
Bibliography: p.
1. Mentally ill—Care—United States—Congresses. I. Menninger, W. Walter. II. Hannah, Gerald T. III. National Conference on the Chronic Mental Patient (2nd : 1984 : Kansas City, Mo.) IV. Title: Chronic mental patient 2. [DNLM: 1. Chronic Disease—congresses. 2. Mental Disorders—congresses. 3. Mental Health Services—United States—congresses. WM 30 C5567 1984]
RC443.C485   1987   362.2'0973   87-1085

ISBN 0-88048-278-8

Contents

Contributors

Leona L. Bachrach, Ph.D.
Associate Professor of Psychiatry,
University of Maryland School of Medicine,
Catonsville, MD

Joseph J. Bevilacqua, Ph.D.
State Commissioner of Mental Health,
Columbia, SC

Neal B. Brown, M.P.A.
Community Support and Rehabilitation Branch,
National Institute of Mental Health,
Rockville, MD

David L. Cutler, M.D.
Associate Professor of Psychiatry,
Oregon Health Sciences University,
Portland, OR

Howard H. Goldman, M.D., Ph.D.
Associate Professor and Director,
Mental Health Policy Studies,
Department of Psychiatry,
University of Maryland School of Medicine,
Baltimore

Gerald T. Hannah, Ph.D.
Commissioner, Kansas State Office of Mental Health
and Retardation Services, Topeka

R. Don Horner, Ph.D.
Program Director,
Kansas Neurological Institute,
Topeka

Judith Katz-Leavy, M.Ed.
Deputy Director,
Child and Adolescent Service System Program,
National Institute of Mental Health,
Rockville, MD

Robert P. Liberman, M.D.
Professor, University of California at Los Angeles School of Medicine;
Director, Clinical Research Center
for Schizophrenia and Psychiatric Rehabilitation,
University of California at Los Angeles

Steve Lyrene, M.D.
Staff Psychiatrist,
Menninger Foundation,
Topeka, KS

Ira S. Lourie, M.D.
Deputy Chief,
Office of State and Community Liaison,
National Institute of Mental Health,
Rockville, MD

Marcia Lovejoy
Former Executive Director,
Project Overcome,
Minneapolis, MN

Ronald W. Manderscheid, Ph.D.
Chief, Survey and Systems Research Branch,
National Institute of Mental Health,
Rockville, MD

W. Walter Menninger, M.D.
Executive Vice President and Chief of Staff,
Menninger Foundation,
Topeka, KS

John H. Noble, Jr., Ph.D.
Professor of Social Work,
State University of New York at Buffalo

Catherine C. Phipps, M.S.
Research Associate,
Clinical Research Center
for Schizophrenia and Psychiatric Rehabilitation,
University of California at Los Angeles School of Medicine

Shirley R. Starr
Co-Founder and Past President,
National Alliance for the Mentally Ill,
Evanston, IL

John A. Talbott, M.D.
Professor and Chairman, Department
of Psychiatry, University of Maryland School of Medicine;
Director, Institute of Psychiatry and Human Behavior,
University of Maryland Medical Systems, Baltimore

Acknowledgments

This book is the result of a national multidisciplinary conference and as such is the product of many people. Our role as organizers and editors was to serve as a catalyst allowing some remarkable persons the opportunity to present and elaborate on their ideas about the plight of the chronically mentally ill. In facilitating this conference and editing this book, we are especially grateful to the following persons and organizations for their assistance and support.

First, the conference owes much to the work of the leadership of and participants in the first National Conference on the Chronic Mental Patient, held in 1978. In particular, we salute the character and dedication of John Talbott, M.D., who spearheaded concern in this area and at the time of this conference was president of the American Psychiatric Association.

Second, we are indebted to the organizations and foundations which identified with our concern and our interest in developing this follow-up conference and provided financial support for it. These are

- the American Psychiatric Association, Melvin Sabshin, M.D., Medical Director, and Corky Hart, Staff Director for the Committee on the Chronically Mentally Ill;
- the National Association of State Mental Health Program Directors, Harry Schnibbe, Executive Director;
- the Menninger Foundation, Roy W. Menninger, President, and Roger Hoffmaster, Administrator, Department of Education;
- the Kansas State Mental Health and Retardation Services, Office of Community Support Programs, Department of Social and Rehabilitation Services;

- the National Institute of Mental Health, Community Support and Rehabilitation Branch; and
- the Marion E. Kenworthy–Sarah H. Swift Foundation, Hon. Justine Wise Polier, President.

Third, the substance of the conference was provided by the careful research and development of ideas in position papers prepared by Howard Goldman, M.D., Ph.D., and Ronald Manderscheid, Ph.D.; Leona Bachrach, Ph.D.; Robert Liberman, M.D., and Catherine Phipps, M.S.; Joseph Bevilacqua, Ph.D., and John Noble, Jr.; Shirley Starr; and Ira Lourie, M.D., and Judith Katz-Leavy, M.Ed. In addition, invaluable were the contributions of John Talbott, M.D., as keynote speaker and Marcia Lovejoy presenting a patient's perspective.

Fourth, the recorders assigned to accompany the formal presenters in the small group discussions helped in numerous ways, not the least of which was in summarizing the discussion at the close of the conference. These were David Cutler, M.D.; Steve Lyrene, M.D.; Arthur Meyerson, M.D.; Neal Brown, M.P.A.; R. Don Horner, Ph.D.; and Blanca Badillo de Loubriel, M.D.

Fifth, our best intentions would mean little in the absence of the support, assistance, and follow-through of our dedicated secretaries, Mary Donohue and Barbara Dyer, who not only handled innumerable logistical details prior to and during the conference, but also labored to help put this book together.

Sixth, in formulating our conclusions, we are grateful for the review and summary of major court decisions in this area as prepared by William Rein, J.D., legal counsel in the Department of Social and Rehabilitation Services for the state of Kansas.

Seventh, we are most appreciative of the support from Ron McMillen and Tim Clancy in accepting our manuscript for publication by the American Psychiatric Press, making it possible for these efforts to reach a broader audience, and from Debbie Klenotic, at the Press, who helped put all the pieces together.

Finally, we thank those concerned professional and lay persons (see Appendix A) who gave up three days of their summer to meet with us in Kansas City and deliberate on these important issues. Their commitment reflects the priority and progress in the mental health field for improving the circumstances and programs for the chronically mentally ill.

W. Walter Menninger, M.D.
Gerald T. Hannah, Ph.D.

Preface

In 1974, a committee of the New York County (Manhattan) District Branch of the American Psychiatric Association drafted an "action paper" on the problems of the care and treatment of the chronic mental patient. Subsequently, that committee and its chairperson, John Talbott, M.D., petitioned the American Psychiatric Association (APA) to undertake a national study of the problem and propose solutions.

John Spiegel, M.D., then president of APA, supported the proposal and utilized his presidential funds to underwrite the work of an APA Ad Hoc Committee on the Chronic Mental Patient, established in 1976. The task of the committee was to plan a national conference on the chronic mental patient. Under Dr. Talbott's leadership, the committee surveyed the membership and committees of APA about problems and possible solutions to the problems presented by and to these patients. The committee reviewed the literature and met with consultants from a wide range of fields—medical economics, medical sociology, health planning, legal rights, legislation, research, and so forth.

Through these efforts, the committee identified seven key questions/issues/topics that were the focus of the first National Conference on the Chronic Mental Patient, held in Washington, D.C., January 11–14, 1978, cosponsored by APA and the President's Commission on Mental Health. Commissioned background papers served as a basis of discussion by the conference participants, with a conference format designed to allow small group discussion of the topics by a wide range of individuals. Finally, the conference papers, discussion, conclusions, and recommendations were assimilated in a report published by APA: *The Chronic Mental Patient: Problems, Solutions, and Recommendations for a Public Policy*.[1]

In 1983, with the burgeoning interest in problems of the chronically mentally ill intensified by the increase of such patients in the community, the time seemed propitious to update the findings of the original conference. It was felt desirable to convene a follow-up conference to bring together new ideas and developments that could be summarized and placed in the hands of mental health practitioners as well as legislators and decision makers. Several concerned organizations—the APA Committee on the Chronically Mentally Ill, the National Association of State Mental Health Program Directors, the National Institute of Mental Health, the Menninger Foundation, and the Kansas State Office of Mental Health and Retardation—were approached to jointly sponsor a small working conference based on a format similar to the first national conference.

This second National Conference on the Chronic Mental Patient was held in Kansas City, Missouri, August 12–14, 1984. As with the earlier conference, papers were commissioned to address key issues and problem areas. Some of these were reassessments of previous problem areas; others looked at new facets not considered in the first conference. These topics were

1. Who are the chronic mentally ill? What changes have we seen in the last 10 years? What trends do we see?
2. Who are the homeless? What are their needs? What trends do we see?
3. What are the innovative treatment techniques in the Community Support Program model that work to meet the needs of clients with chronic mental illness?
4. What are the obstacles to implementing programs for the chronically mentally ill? What are the financial and control issues in providing services for the chronic mentally ill (state versus federal)? What are the legal issues associated with providing services for the chronic mentally ill? What are the problems associated with societal stereotypes of persons with chronic mental illness?
5. What is the role of families and ex-patients in providing care and support for the chronic mentally ill client?
6. Who are the children with chronic mental illness? What are they? What are these children's needs and their rights?

---

[1]Talbott JA (Ed): The Chronic Mental Patient: Problems, Solutions, and Recommendations for a Public Policy. Washington, DC, American Psychiatric Association, 1978

In addition to the discussion papers, two additional perspectives were sought. To keynote the gathering, Dr. Talbott, then president of APA, shared with the conferees his perspective on the problem. He drew on his experience with the original New York District Branch Committee and the APA Ad Hoc Committee on the Chronic Mental Patient, which he chaired until he assumed the APA presidency. During the conference, Marcia Lovejoy, executive director of Project Overcome in Minneapolis, Minnesota, and an acknowledged "non-practicing schizophrenic" presented an articulate view from the perspective of a former patient.

This volume represents the work product of this second national conference. It is intended as a follow-up and supplement to the report of the 1978 conference. As with that report, this document follows the format of the conference, beginning with the keynote address and a patient's perspective, followed by the six background papers. These papers have been edited by the presenters to incorporate some of the conference discussion. A final substantive chapter is offered by the editors with a summary of conclusions and recommendations drawn from the various papers and discussions. In the appendixes are details of the conference agenda and participants; additional observations by recorders summarizing discussion of four of the topics; relevant position papers and statements; and some additional suggested readings on the subject of the chronic mentally ill.

As noted above, this report, like this conference, is not intended to duplicate or supplant the work of the first national conference. Rather, it is intended to supplement and expand that work. Persons interested in a full picture of the issues, problems, and proposed solutions to the plight of these patients should therefore study the 1978 Conference Report as well as this one.

As with the earlier report, this publication is another step in the implementation of public policy to improve the care and conditions of chronic mentally ill persons. Its purpose will be best served if it becomes the basis for continued discussion and action by professional organizations; social action coalitions; organizations of ex-patients and families of mentally ill; and governmental bodies on the local, state, and federal levels. The organizers, supporters, and participants of this conference did not want their efforts to end in the meeting rooms of the conference site. Rather, they felt these ideas should be reproduced and disseminated widely, to the ultimate benefit of those many emotionally troubled persons who do not have the capacity or forum for articulating their own needs and concerns.

CHAPTER 1

The Chronic Mentally Ill: What Do We Now Know, and Why Aren't We Implementing What We Know?

JOHN A. TALBOTT, M.D.

In 1978 most of the data were collected that constituted the reports on the chronic mentally ill that were subsequently published by the American Psychiatric Association (APA) (1), the Group for the Advancement of Psychiatry (GAP) (2), and the President's Commission on Mental Health (3). Since then, a great deal of research and study has been conducted on this population. It has provided us with a good deal of new information about the treatment and care of this population that we did not then know. In this contribution I will summarize what we now know, emphasizing what is new (4) since the publication of the three pivotal reports (1–3), then discuss why we are not implementing what we know, and conclude with some predictions for the future.

Before I proceed, I wish to define the population I am talking about. I, as well as APA's Committee on the Chronically Mentally Ill, have found most useful the definition offered by Bachrach (5); to wit, those people who are or might have been in public mental hospitals, especially state hospitals, 30 years ago. Therefore, I am not using the term only for those suffering from a particular illness, only for those who have been discharged from state facilities, or only for those of a specific age group. The chronic mentally ill include those suffering from severe, episodic, and chronic mental illnesses; the 30 percent of new admissions to programs in the community serving the chronically ill who have never been hospitalized; and both children (who constitute four percent of the population) and the elderly (whose rate of mental illness increases exponentially after the age of 65). For reasons of simplicity, the definition does not, however, include the mentally retarded or those suffering from alcohol or drug abuse.

WHAT WE NOW KNOW

As I mentioned above, in 1978 we did know several important things about the chronic mentally ill (5). We knew something about their numbers, location, functioning, and needs. In addition, we knew about a number of model programs for the chronically ill, as well as what factors ensured continuing treatment in the community. Finally, we knew something about the economic factors that controlled treatment and care of the chronic mentally ill and something about cost/benefit studies.

However, in the past 8 years the amount of information we have accumulated about the chronic mentally ill is greater than that published over the entire past 80 years. As an illustration, the appendix of the 1978 APA publication on the chronic mentally ill gave only 46 references. In this section I will summarize some of the new data regarding 1) the population, 2) treatment and care, and 3) program principles.

Population

In 1978 we knew that the number of chronic mentally ill persons in the United States was large (estimated between 1 and 7 million), but it took the National Institute of Mental Health's (NIMH's) study (6) to specify that we had 3 million persons suffering from severe mental illnesses, 2.4 million who had had these illnesses for a long time (that is, were chronic) and 1.7 million who not only had been suffering for a long time but had resultant disability (see Figure 1).

Where do these 1.7 million severely and chronically mentally ill and disabled individuals reside? As we know, the nationwide peak in state hospital census was achieved in 1955. Since then the state hospital population has steadily, and in the late 1960s, precipitously, declined and now has essentially bottomed out (see Figure 2).

Those persons who remain in state facilities consist of two large groups: 1) those 65 and over who have been and will be hospitalized for lengthy periods, and 2) a much younger (thirtyish) group who come into the hospital for much shorter periods of time (see Figure 3).

For these younger individuals, the hospital is but one small portion of their treatment and living experience. Readmission rates to state facilities have changed dramatically since 1955. Over 60 percent of all

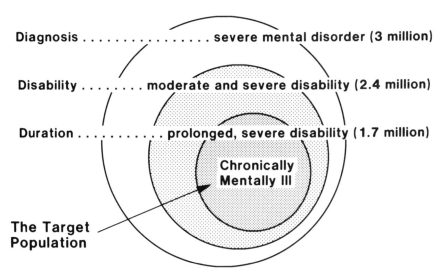

Figure 1. The estimated number of chronically mentally ill. From the National Plan for the Chronically Mentally Ill.

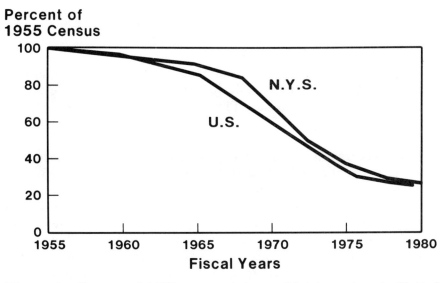

Figure 2. Percent of 1955 census state psychiatric centers in United States and New York. From New York State Office of Mental Health, 1981.

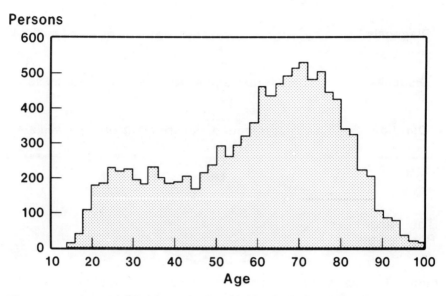

Figure 3.   Age profile of residents of New York State psychiatric hospitals.

admissions now are readmissions, and all discharged patients have about a 60 percent change of being readmitted within a 2-year period (see Figure 4).

Since state hospitals, which contained 560,000 chronic mentally ill patients in 1955, now contain only 130,000 such persons, where else do the chronic mentally ill reside? First and foremost, they live in other institutions, primarily nursing homes. Indeed, since the percentage of Americans in all types of institutions did not change between 1950 and 1970, it is apparent that what was experienced could more aptly be termed transinstitutionalization than deinstitutionalization (see Figure 5).

While state hospital populations underwent a decline to one-third of their previous size, the size of nursing home populations trebled. This presents us with a massive public policy problem in the next few years with the continuing "greying of America." We know that the population over the age of 65 will double by the year 2030, that mental illness increases dramatically in this group, and that 50 percent of nursing home beds are now occupied with persons suffering from mental illness. Thus, if states continue to place a freeze on construction of new nursing home beds, there will be no logical institution in which to care for the elderly mentally ill who no longer need acute hospital care (see Figure 6).

Aside from the vast numbers of persons who were transinstitutionalized to nursing homes, it is obvious from the picture seen in all too many urban communities that a large number of young, chronic mentally

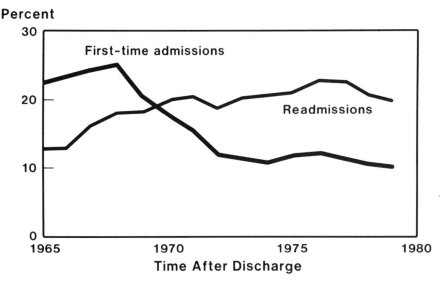

Figure 4. Admission and readmission rates for New York State psychiatric hospitals.

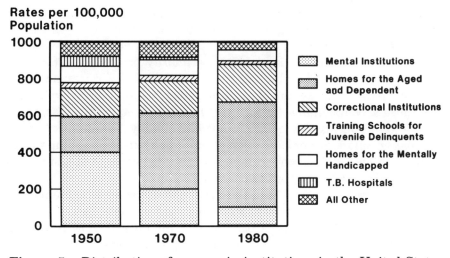

Figure 5. Distribution of persons in institutions in the United States per 100,000 population by type of institution. From U.S. Bureau of the Census.

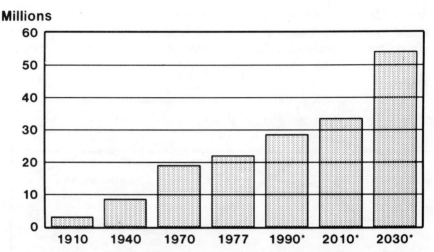

Figure 6. Estimates of Americans over age 65. *Assumes a fertility rate of 2.1 children born per woman and a decreasing mortality rate such that life expectancy at birth increases by about .05 year per year.

ill individuals have (as it were) overflowed into our cities' streets. They are the visible evidence of the huge post World War II baby boom population, which only now is aging into the decades in which they will either develop symptoms of schizophrenia or come into contact with the health system for its treatment (see Figure 7).

These "new" or young chronic mentally ill individuals have been the subject of great concern in the field, primarily because of their overwhelming numbers, their high degree of utilization of services, and their noncompliance with treatment (up to 83 percent) (7, 8). They are generally described as young males (20–35) who have no permanent homes, abuse substances frequently, have high arrest rates (mainly for "nuisance" crimes or misdemeanors rather than felonies) and high suicide rates (up to four percent in one study), poor social and vocational skills, and histories of violent behavior or poor impulse control.

Some have clearly entered the correctional system. The numbers of those housed in prisons and jails who have mental illness, as well as those who are in mental hospitals because of criminal behavior, have both increased beyond the increase experienced by the prison system in general (see Figure 8).

While the needs of the chronic mentally ill have been known for a long time, it is only relatively recently that we have had a comprehensive conceptualization of how those needs are met in different types of settings.

Elizabeth Boggs has placed human needs along the horizontal axis and settings along the vertical axis, in descending order of restrictiveness, to give us a schema that enables us to see readily the range of settings needed to house this population. It is clear that in moving from a total

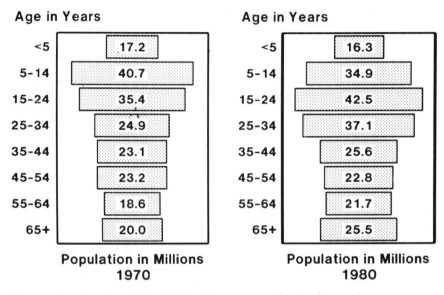

Figure 7. Profile of the United States population by age group.

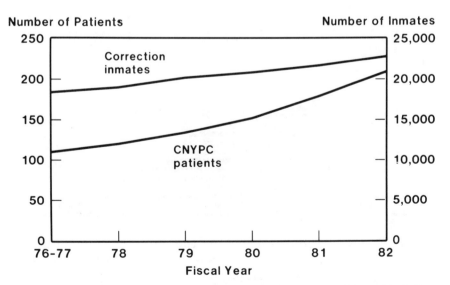

Figure 8. New York State forensic population: City of New York Psychiatric Center and corrections institutions.

institution to an independent living setting, one's needs in no way diminish and some means must be found to fulfill those needs not met in any particular setting (see Figure 9).

From such a realization, it is also clear that hospitals are but one part of the total picture (see Figure 10).

Treatment and Care

Since 1978 there have also been advances in understanding how best to treat and care for the chronically ill. I have divided these into the areas of knowledge about systems of care, hospital versus community care, hospital care alone, community care alone, disease processes, rehabilitation, and economic issues.

In terms of what we have learned about systems of care, there are two new important items. First, it is clear both from the Boggs schema and existing programmatic models that the chronic mentally ill must have a range of settings and services available (see Figure 11).

Second, as the Veterans Administration Collaborative Day Hospital Study (9) demonstrated, continuity of care may be far more important that any other single treatment or care ingredient. In addition, the pertinent studies on what prevents or forestalls both hospitalization and exacerbation of illness reveal the fact that the two most potent weapons

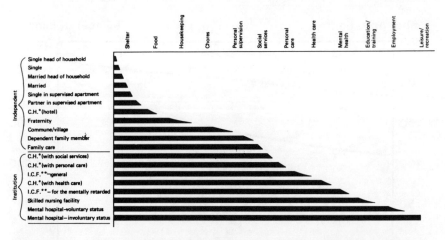

Figure 9. Needs and settings for the chronically mentally ill. C.H. = congregate housing; I.C.F. = intermediate care facility. From Elizabeth Boggs, Ph.D., personal communication, 1984.

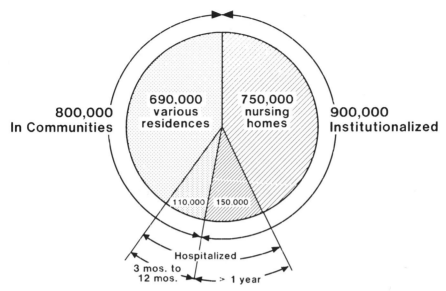

Figure 10. The location of the chronically mentally ill in the United States in 1977. From the National Plan for the Chronically Mentally Ill.

we have in our armamentarium are 1) continuing medication and 2) continued personal contact (for example, psychotherapy). If that is the case, then the facts that fewer than 50 percent of discharged patients continue to take their prescribed medication and only 25 percent continue in some form of outpatient care (for example, aftercare) lead to the inescapable conclusion that continuity of care is of paramount importance to insure the provision of those few treatment elements that work for the chronic mentally ill (10).

Regarding the controversy over whether it is better to treat the chronic mentally ill in a hospital or in a community setting, there have been several reviews of the literature on these alternatives. The most recent of these, by Kiesler (11) and Braun et al. (12), reach essentially the same conclusion—that there is no advantage to hospital care and, indeed, some advantage to community care (for example, improvement of symptomatology and quality of life), including the fact that individuals like it better. This is not to say, however, that we will not always need hospitals for some segment of the mentally ill who need ongoing supervision, high degrees of structure, and limits placed on their impulsivity or confused wanderings. However, experts agree that the percentage of such individuals is probably only about two to three percent, and such settings, while

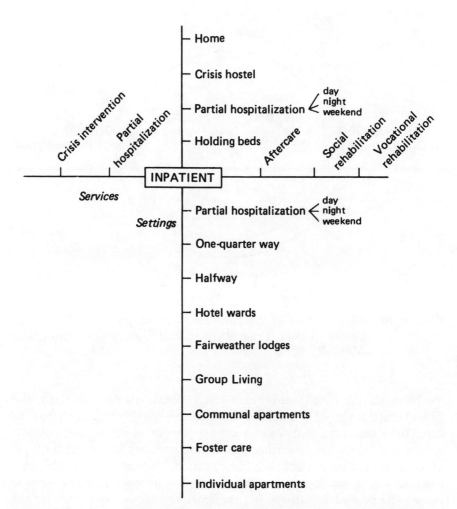

Figure 11. The ranges of settings (vertical axis) and services (horizontal axis) that must be available to one chronic mental patient.

offering asylum, in no way need to be traditional state-run asylums (13). Indeed, they can be small, locked facilities located in the community, modeled along the lines of intermediary care facilities. Such programs, pioneered in California, called "L-facilities," are considered by many experts to be far superior to either hospitals or unsupervised community residences for a specific defined subset of the chronic mentally ill (14).

Regarding hospital treatment, a recent article by Glick et al. (15) concludes that whereas for first-break schizophrenics lengthy hospitalizations are preferable, for the chronic mentally ill brief readmissions for reequilibration of their medication and reformulation of their treatment plan, followed by prompt return to a community support system, are optimal. Our training and thinking, however, still tend to dictate short-term hospital stays for those suffering from acute illnesses and longer-term stays for chronic patients.

Several states, notably New York and Texas, have conducted studies of their state hospital populations and concluded that one-third of their patients would not need that level of care *if* an adequate number of community alternatives were available, and one-third could live in the community *if* a good community support system were available. The hitch is the ifs—we have neither enough alternatives nor enough good community support programs, despite NIMH's eight years of energetic activity in this arena.

With respect to community care for the chronic mentally ill, there are several developments that have direct bearing on better treatment and care for this population. First, it now appears that while medication and psychosocial interventions are not additive, they are interactive, and neither is sufficient in and of itself (16). Second, while adequate doses of medication are essential for symptom suppression in the acute phase or during acute exacerbations of chronic illness, they are often detrimental after the discharge when patients' coping skills need honing (17). Third, from May's and others' work, it is reasonable to conclude that for the chronically ill in the community, group therapy has the edge over individual treatment (18).

In regard to what we now know about the serious diseases commonly found among the chronic mentally ill, there are also many new developments. Foremost among these is the completion of several long-term follow-up studies of schizophrenics, both in this country and abroad (19–22). These studies are revealing in many ways: they demonstrate that schizophrenia has many courses, and indeed most commonly results in either recovery or mild outcomes; that only 40 percent of persons afflicted will have a bad outcome; and that onset, course, and outcome are independent (see Figure 12). These data are especially useful in advising families of schizophrenics that their relatives' futures are not inevitably bleak.

In addition, the work of Herz (23), as well as that of Carpenter et al. (24), demonstrates that early signs and symptoms of relapse can be identified for both schizophrenics as a group and individuals suffering from the disorder. This is terribly important clinically, since with use of intermittent or low-dose schedules of medications, patients and families can be taught to be on the alert for signs of exacerbations of illness, permitting prompt and aggressive reintroduction of psychotropics.

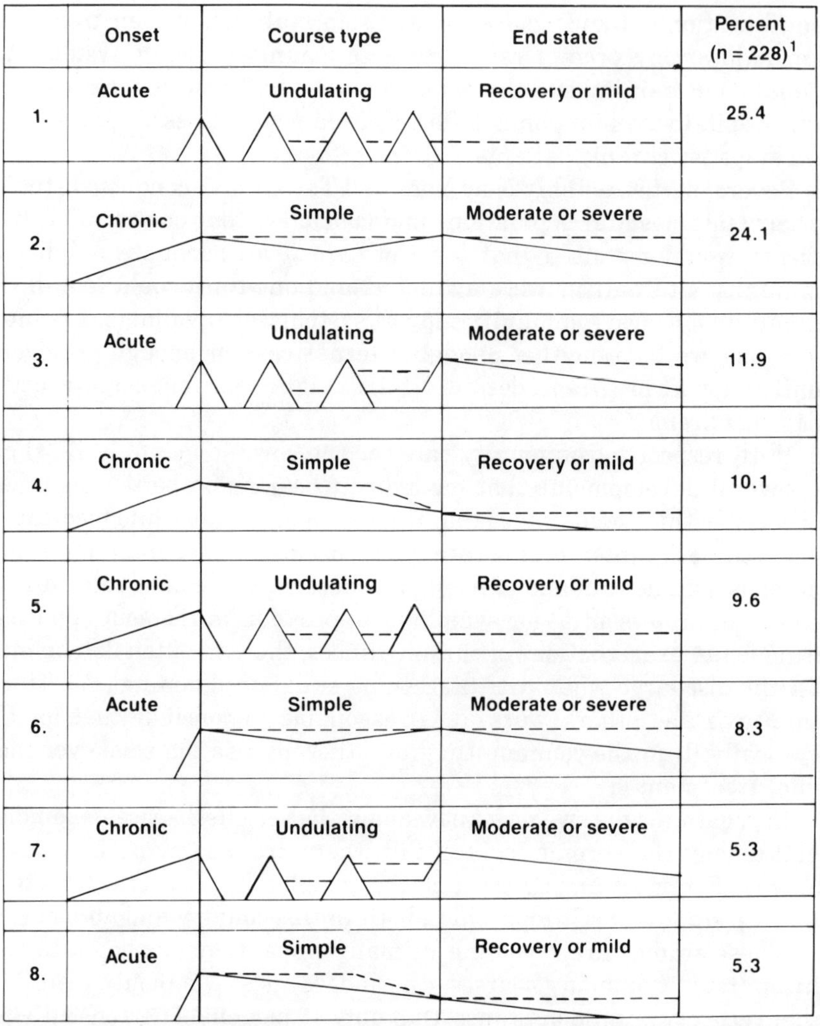

	Onset	Course type	End state	Percent (n = 228)[1]
1.	Acute	Undulating	Recovery or mild	25.4
2.	Chronic	Simple	Moderate or severe	24.1
3.	Acute	Undulating	Moderate or severe	11.9
4.	Chronic	Simple	Recovery or mild	10.1
5.	Chronic	Undulating	Recovery or mild	9.6
6.	Acute	Simple	Moderate or severe	8.3
7.	Chronic	Undulating	Moderate or severe	5.3
8.	Acute	Simple	Recovery or mild	5.3

Figure 12.   Long-term outcome for persons suffering from schizophrenia.

[1]In 61 cases of 289 (21.1 percent), onset, course type, or end state could not be determined with certainty.

Another terribly important therapeutic development concerns the introduction of so-called psychoeducational approaches with families and patients (25, 26). All these programs are essentially based on the original work by investigators in the United Kingdom (27), which demonstrated that the relapse rates for schizophrenics living with families exhibiting high expressed emotion (EE) but on medication was about the same as those living with low EE families without medication (see Figure 13). They utilize this information and attempt to teach patients and families about the disease process, treatment approaches, and most importantly, about how to reduce intrafamilial stress. In addition they seek to avoid "blaming the family" and instead emphasize working together to achieve the best outcome possible. The results are extremely encouraging, demonstrating that patients involved in such efforts have one-third to one-eighth the readmission rates of their controls.

We also know much more now about rehabilitation of the chronically ill. For instance, we know that the severity of a person's disease state is not related to the degree of his or her disability; for example, a person can be very sick but less disabled or vice versa (28). Second, we now realize from the work of Strauss and Carpenter (29) that individual elements only predict themselves; for example, previous vocational functioning only predicts future vocational functioning, not future social functioning, symptomatology, and so forth. Lastly, we know now that an individual person's level of disability depends more on his or her skills and activity than on his or her psychopathology (30).

A final area involving treatment and care that we know much more about today than in 1978 concerns economics. From several comparisons (31–35) of the cost of community care versus hospital care several conclusions can be drawn. First, both forms of care for this population are costly—over $7,200 a year for community care or hospital treatment plus traditional aftercare (31). However, it should be noted that any comparison of community with institutional care assumes we have only one or

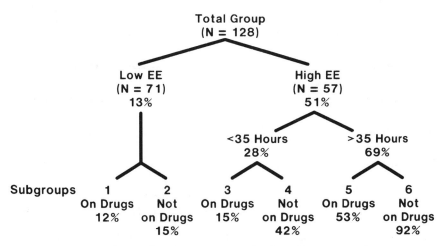

Figure 13. Nine-month relapse rates of schizophrenic patients.

the other, whereas we are essentially funding at least two competing systems of care. Thus, unless we abolish one or the other, we are "double-funding" our delivery system (see Figure 14).

Second, states do save money, some 65–80 percent, each time a patient is deinstitutionalized, since state hospital funding comes almost 100 percent from state tax levy monies, whereas community care is financed mainly by federal and local funding (for example, Medicaid, Medicare, and Supplemental Security Income [SSI]) (32). Third, while there is some cost-saving with community care, it is not great. And finally, while we have greatly expanded the outpatient services available in America, their presence has not decreased the number of episodes of mental illness treated on inpatient services (see Figure 15).

Principles of Successful Programs

From a variety of reviews (33–35) it is possible to construct a list of elements deemed essential to successful programs serving the chronic mentally ill. These include:

- offering lifetime access to a range of comprehensive services (for example, replacing all the services available in a hospital with the same range of services in the community under a single "umbrella");
- treating hospitalization as only one part of the totality of services needed by this population, but ensuring that it is indeed available;

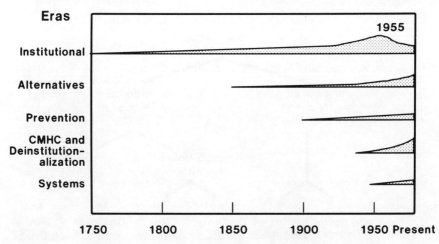

Figure 14. Phases of development of mental health services. (CMHC = community mental health center)

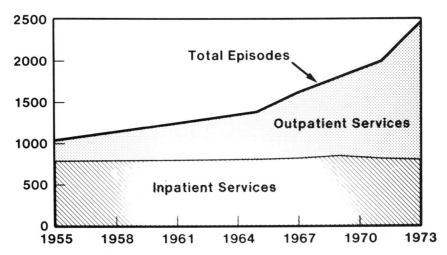

Figure 15. Patient–care episodes per 100,000 population.

- treating each episode of illness or treatment as only one part of a patient's entire lifetime risk for illness and need for availability of treatment;
- providing all the services available in the traditional hospital in an assertive manner, for example, by going out actively and engaging reluctant patients;
- targeting the chronic mentally ill population as a primary object of care rather than seeing it as undesirable or consisting of "second-rate teaching cases";
- feeling accountable for care delivered to this population and actually being held accountable;
- performing internal evaluation as to how successful the program is in meeting its goals;
- being culturally relevant; that is, not only taking into account racial, religious, and other factors but what resources already exist in the community;
- providing a true community support system;
- ensuring continuity of care by case management or resource linkage;
- providing both psychosocial and psychopharmacologic interventions together;
- utilizing skilled personnel and providing them with specialized training;
- focusing on the training of patients in survival skills; that is, the skills of everyday living.

WHY CAN'T WE DO WHAT WE KNOW WORKS?

If after a decade of intense work with the chronic mentally ill, we know as much as we do about the population—their optimal treatment and care and principles of successful programs—why hasn't this knowledge been successfully translated into action? Essentially, there are seven reasons: attitudes, economic factors, governmental structure, lack of responsibility for care, people problems, legal and regulatory constraints, and research trends. Each will be summarized below.

Attitudes

It is hard to think of a group of "have-nots" in America that has less public sympathy, less lobbying clout, and a lower priority for funding than the chronic mentally ill. The negative attitudes that affect the chronically ill are held by both community leaders and caregivers. Community leaders want fairly simple and time-limited solutions rather than recommendations for more long-term care; the public still senses that the mentally ill are at least partially to blame for their illness (contrasted to the mentally retarded, whose families have successfully destigmatized themselves over the past 25 years); and the chronically ill, with no lobbying clout, little power of taxation, and even weaker voting power, have insufficient voice to demand otherwise. Unfortunately, when caregivers lobby, they are often seen as self-serving; therefore, it is extremely useful when groups such as the National Alliance for the Mentally Ill advocate for improved services.

Caregivers have somewhat different attitudinal problems. Most physicians enter medical school with a desire to cure patients, not merely care for them; psychiatry is one of the few specialties where the most-skilled practitioners take care of the least-impaired patients; many in the field express the opinion that care of the chronically ill is neither "sexy" nor "interesting" (as if we became physicians to be entertained); and there are very few rewards or thank-you's from the chronically ill.

The reasons for these negative attitudes about the chronically ill are both neurotic and realistic. They are neurotic in that some people are still afraid of "catching" mental illness from its sufferers or fear the emergence of the "little bit of craziness in us all." Realistic feelings stem, however, from the fact that neither institutional nor community programs for the chronically ill have covered themselves with glory in the past 200 years, and the population is a terribly difficult one to treat and maintain interest in.

Economic Factors

The economic barriers to effecting good care and treatment of the chronic mentally ill are also impressive. First, we have no single system of care in this nation. Instead, we have multiple systems, each competing for the same patients and resources: for example, public (Public Health Service, Veterans Administration, community mental health centers [CMHCs], state hospital, county hospital, and so forth); quasi-public (university and voluntary not-for-profit institutions); and private individual and "chain" hospitals. In addition, with the establishment of each new subsystem, additional costs are generated. Second, each level of government (federal, state, and local) has an inherent conflict of interest between operating its own facilities and contracting with community agencies, and in times of scarcity will direct community-designated monies to back-flow into their own facilities to save them. Third, services are financed by per diem (for inpatient) and fee-for-service (for outpatient care) mechanisms rather than capitation, encouraging inpatient admissions rather than preventive services and maintenance in the community. Fourth, as stated above, through the provision of federal Medicaid, Medicare, and SSI monies, states were able to shift the economic burden for patients in state hospitals from almost 100 percent state tax levy monies to largely federal funding (with some local sharing). The result was that while patients moved out, resources did not, tied as they were to state hospital beds (see Figure 16).

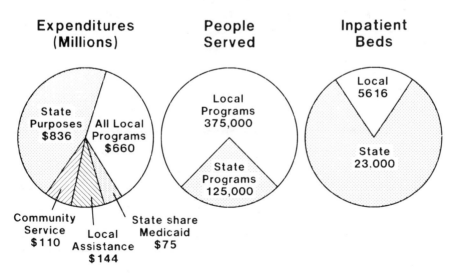

Figure 16. New York State state and local program shares.

The total bill in 1974 for psychiatric care in this nation was approximately $37 billion (see Figure 17). About half of this money went for direct services, and the remainder went for indirect ones (for example, loss of service, loss of product, and so forth). If we recall that there are fewer than three million chronic mentally ill persons in this country, simple division reveals that each person accounts for about $10,000 a year, a not-inconsiderable sum when compared with the figure of $7,200/year needed for good community care given by Stein et al. (31).

When direct services (that is, those paid to providers) are examined, it is apparent why the percentage of monies allocatable to the chronic mentally ill is so high—87 percent or $32 billion of the $37 billion. It is because a sizable proportion, over 50 percent, goes to nursing homes and state and county hospitals, while a relatively small percentage goes to general hospitals (11 percent) and CMHCs (4 percent) (see Figure 18).

Current reimbursement systems have incentives and disincentives that are almost completely the reverse of those needed to bring about better community care for the chronically mentally ill. They reward

- more restrictive rather than less restrictive settings;
- public rather than private facilities (for example, in New York, the same physician seeing a patient in a hospital clinic is paid twice what he would receive seeing the same patient in his private office, which has much lower overhead costs);
- acute rather than chronic care;
- the promise of cure rather than the pursuit of care;
- inpatient admission rather than maintenance in the community; and
- direct services (for example, contact) rather than indirect ones (for example, coordinating with other agencies and professionals).

In addition, most services needed by the chronic mentally ill are financed piecemeal rather than comprehensively, and some funding (for

Cost	1963	1968	1971	1974	1980
Direct	2,402	4,031	11,058	16,973	23,558
Indirect	4,634	16,906	14,179	19,813	28,860
Total	7,036	20,937	25,238	36,786	52,418

Figure 17. Estimated total costs of mental illness in the United States (in millions).

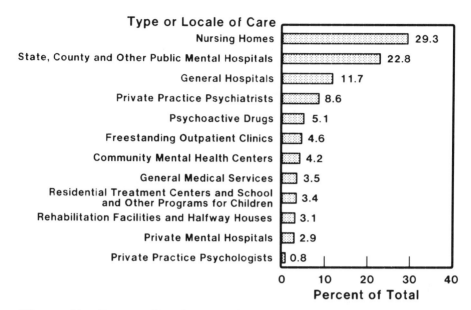

Figure 18. Percent distribution of expenditures for direct care of the mentally ill by type or locale of care: United States, 1974. From Statistical Note No. 125, Division of Biometry and Epidemiology, National Institute of Mental Health.

example, nursing home funding via social service channels) is totally inaccessible to mental health officials seeking to improve these facilities. Finally, to date, no region in the country has found a mechanism to fund asylums or to adequately provide low-cost accessible housing alternatives for this population.

Governmental Structure

As mentioned above, there is no genuine system of care in this country. Instead, if one tried to draw a table of organization of the "system" it would resemble Figure 19. The resultant system invites political fights between all of its elements and, as stated before, has inherent conflicts of interest at each level of government.

In addition, almost every need identified for the chronically ill is met by a different federal and state agency (see Figure 20).

Because of differing legislative mandates, each agency has differing requirements for funding and differing ideas of who it is serving. The result is overwhelming fragmentation, with multiple streams of funds,

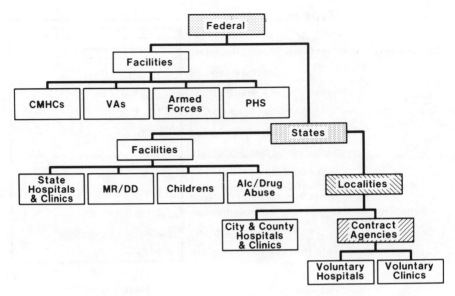

Figure 19. Levels of government funding of psychiatric care. CMHC = community mental health center; VA = Veterans Administration; PHS = Public Health Service; MR/DD = Mental Retardation/Developmental Disability.

multiple levels of planning, and multiple loci of implementation. All too often, these streams of funding come down separately, without any attempt to pull them together into an accessible package to meet real live patients' needs rather than bureaucratic ideals (see Figure 21).

Housing	Income	Vocational Rehab	Social Rehab	Medical	Psychiatric
(HUD)	(SSI)	(HRA)	(HSA)	(Medicaid/ Medicare)	(CMHC/State /Local)

Figure 20. Needs of the chronically mentally ill and who meets them. HUD = U.S. Department of Housing and Urban Development; SSI = Supplemental Security Income; HRA = Human Resources Administration; HSA = Health Services Administration; CMHC = community mental health center.

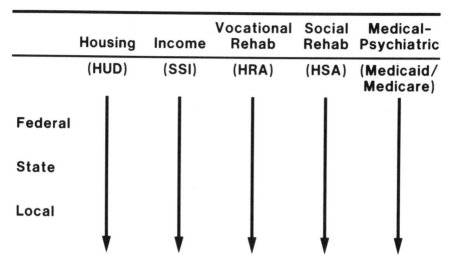

	Housing	Income	Vocational Rehab	Social Rehab	Medical– Psychiatric
	(HUD)	(SSI)	(HRA)	(HSA)	(Medicaid/ Medicare)
Federal					
State					
Local					

Figure 21. The many separate streams of funding for mental health care in the United States. HUD = U.S. Department of Housing and Urban Development; SSI = Supplemental Security Income; HRA = Human Resources Administration; HSA = Health Services Administration.

Responsibility

In moving from a single system (the state hospital) to multiple settings in the community, our ability to pinpoint the responsibility for care of both the entire population and individual patients was lost. To regain this most essential ingredient of good care, "point responsibility" must be reestablished for each patient (see Figure 22); each group of patients (see Figure 23); and the entire population of the chronic mentally ill (see Figure 24).

Essentially, no one is in charge at present—a situation that causes endless numbers of problems.

People Problems

Barriers to more effective care and treatment of the chronically ill are also posed by several groups, including program administrators, staff members, unions, and average citizens. Leaders of programs serving the chronic mentally ill must understand the process of chronicity, be interested in persons suffering from chronic conditions, and be able to walk that fine line between expecting too much of patients, prompting their

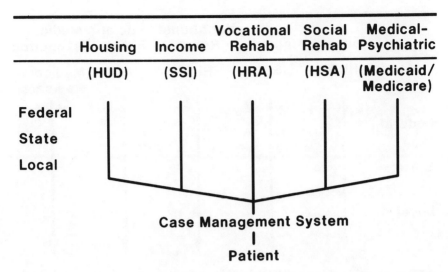

	Housing	Income	Vocational Rehab	Social Rehab	Medical-Psychiatric
	(HUD)	(SSI)	(HRA)	(HSA)	(Medicaid/Medicare)
Federal					
State					
Local					

Case Management System

Patient

Figure 22. How responsibility should be pinpointed in the treatment of each patient. HUD = U.S. Department of Housing and Urban Development; SSI = Supplemental Security Income; HRA = Human Resources Administration; HSA = Health Services Administration.

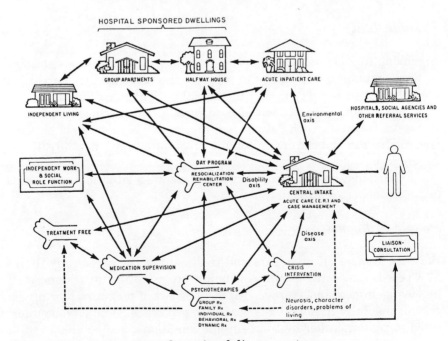

Figure 23. An integrated service delivery system.

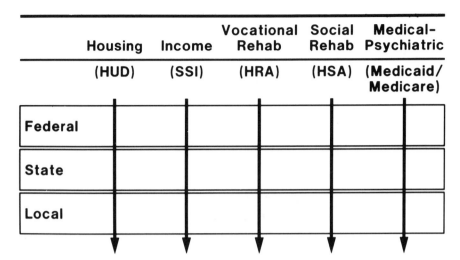

	Housing	Income	Vocational Rehab	Social Rehab	Medical-Psychiatric
	(HUD)	(SSI)	(HRA)	(HSA)	(Medicaid/ Medicare)
Federal					
State					
Local					

Figure 24. How responsibility should be pinpointed in the treatment of the entire population of the chronically mentally ill. HUD = Department of Housing and Urban Development; SSI = Supplemental Security Income; HRA = Human Resources Administration; HSA = Health Services Administration.

regression, and holding up enough hope to encourage attainment of higher levels of functioning. Staff members must recognize this same balance and have exposure to and training in modern resocialization-relearning approaches, effective rehabilitation techniques to remedy disabilities, teaching patients in the skills of everyday living, and psychoeducational approaches with both patients and families.

Unions of employees from the governmental sector also present a sizable obstacle to the move toward community care. In New York State, new monies for mental health have gone in recent years into bringing the ratio of patients to staff to 1:1, a ratio that was promised by the most recent governor, then running for reelection, to the civil service union, before any monies could be reallocated to community settings (see Figure 25). In addition, many communities in which state hospitals are located have strenuously resisted reallocation of resources because of their dependence on these facilities for jobs, business, and so forth.

Legal and Regulatory Pressures

The judicial findings, governmental regulations, and legal developments in the past few decades, designed to remedy the very real abuse that

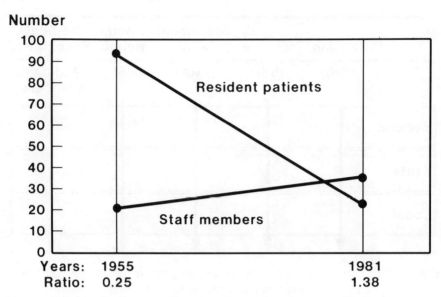

Figure 25.   Ratio of resident patients to staff of New York State psychiatric centers.

indeed existed in some facilities, have often hampered quality care for the chronically ill. For instance, *Souder v. Brennan*, intended to remedy the abuse of peonage of state patients, instead resulted in the closure of thousands of legitimate work programs. Likewise, the multiplicity of standards promulgated by the Joint Commission on the Accreditation of Hospitals and other regulatory bodies, while attempting to provide guidelines for ensuring quality of care, have often merely focused attention on what can be measured easily rather than clinical outcome or program success. In addition, the sheer number of agencies (164 in New York State)—national, state, and local—that can come into any hospital, inspect it, and require new forms to be filled out drives care toward paper compliance rather than clinical excellence (see Figure 26). In New York, it has been calculated that 25 percent of all staff time and 25 percent of a hospital's resources go toward complying with regulatory agency standards—in addition to providing good care, accurate medical records, and so forth (36).

Research Trends

Given the current excitement in our field about the promising developments in basic research that will hopefully soon illuminate the underlying

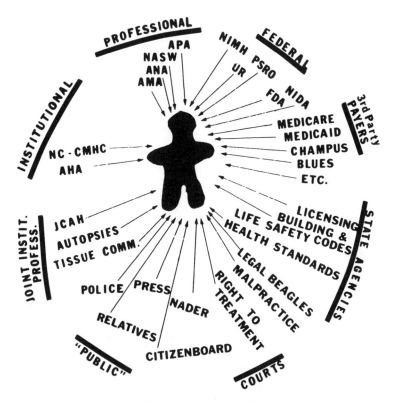

Figure 26. The various agencies that can impose standards on a hospital. APA = American Psychiatric Association; NASW = National Association of Social Workers; ANA = American Nurses' Association; AMA = American Medical Association; NC-CMHC = National Council of Community Mental Health Centers; AHA = American Hospital Association; JCAH = Joint Commission on Accreditation of Hospitals; UR = Utilization Review; NIMH/PSRO = professional standards; FDA = U.S. Food and Drug Administration; NIDA = National Institute of Drug Abuse; CHAMPUS = Civilian Health and Medical Program for Uniformed Services.

etiology of the major mental illnesses, the future of effective treatment of the chronic mentally ill may indeed hinge on basic science breakthroughs. However, while awaiting these breakthroughs, it is critical to focus attention on several unanswered questions important to the care and treatment of the chronically ill. These include:

- What causes and prevents chronicity?
- What treatment elements work for which patients in what settings?
- How many of each setting and service do we need, how much do they cost, and how do we provide enough of them (especially asylum settings)?

WHAT DO WE DO NOW?

It is my prediction that given the current political climate, economic trends, and governmental social, mental health, and housing policies, things will get worse for the chronic mentally ill before they get better. I fear that the numbers of the homeless will continue to rise; that prison populations of the mentally ill will swell; and that both community (for example, nursing homes) and institutional (for example, state hospitals) scandals will become more common.

We have already heard scattered cries for rehospitalization (from, among others, the editors of *The New York Times*), and these will no doubt be heard again. But given the vast monies necessary, not only to rebuild the deteriorating plants in our public facilities but to bring about effective reform of the public system—as well as the fact that reinstitutionalization would fly in the face of the last 25 years of scientific study and legal pressure—its actualization is unlikely.

On the other hand, there may be renewed calls to close state hospitals and move entirely to a community care system for the chronically ill. Certainly, the Massachusetts Blue Ribbon Commission report calls for this direction (37).

Instead of these outcomes, it is my opinion that we will move to a reallocation of resources and redivision of labor among the disparate parts of the mental health system (38).

One way of conceptualizing a new breakdown of functions of the traditional state facility is to divide asylum, treatment, and care elements, all of which should be supported by state funding, but any of which can be provided in community settings.

HOW CAN THIS BE ACCOMPLISHED?

There are several methods by which a move toward reallocation of resources and redivision of labor could be achieved. They include:

1. Capitation funding, as in Wisconsin (39), which rewards prevention, alternatives to hospitalization, and community care.
2. Health maintenance organization or prepaid medical service programs that also promote prevention, continuity of care, and indirect services.

3. A voucher system that would provide each chronically mentally ill person in America one voucher for housing and another for services.
4. Changes in current reimbursement mechanisms so that day hospitals, psychosocial rehabilitation programs, and other alternatives to inpatient hospitalization are more adequately reimbursed than inpatient care itself.
5. A truly unified system that would incorporate all elements of our disparate mental health system.
6. More money for the chronic mentally ill.

At this point, it is impossible to predict what we, as a nation, will choose to do with our disjointed, ineffective, and inefficient mental health services. But given the crunch occasioned by the huge numbers of new young chronic mentally ill persons and rapidly increasing numbers of older persons suffering from mental illness, we are at a critical point. What we do will reveal not only our ingenuity but our ability to act humanely in the best interests of those who do not and cannot speak effectively for themselves.

REFERENCES

1. Talbott JA (ed): The Chronic Mental Patient: Problems, Solutions, and Recommendations for a Public Policy. Washington, DC, American Psychiatric Association, 1978
2. Group for the Advancement of Psychiatry: The Chronic Mental Patient in the Community. New York, Group for the Advancement of Psychiatry, 1978
3. President's Commission on Mental Health: Report to the President. Washington, DC, U.S. Government Printing Office, 1978
4. Talbott JA (ed): The Chronic Mental Patient: Five Years Later. Orlando, FL, Grune and Stratton, 1984
5. Bachrach LL: Deinstitutionalization: An Analytical Review and Sociological Perspective. Rockville, MD, National Institute of Mental Health, 1976
6. Talbott JA: Toward a public policy on the chronically mentally ill. Am J Orthopsychiatry 50:43–53, 1980
7. Pepper B, Ryglewicz H (eds): The Young Adult Chronic Patient. New Directions for Mental Health Services, no. 14. San Francisco, Jossey-Bass, 1982
8. Pepper B, Ryglewicz H (eds): Advances in Treating the Young Adult Chronic Patient. New Directions for Mental Health Services, no. 21. San Francisco, Jossey-Bass, 1984

9. Linn MW, Caffey EM, Klett CJ, et al: Day treatment and psychotropic drugs in the aftercare of schizophrenic patients. Arch Gen Psychiatr 36:1055–1072, 1979

10. Minkoff K: A map of chronic mental patients, in The Chronic Mental Patient: Problems, Solutions, and Recommendations for a Public Policy. Edited by Talbott JA. Washington, DC, American Psychiatric Association, 1978

11. Kiesler CA: Mental hospitals and alternative care: noninstitutionalization as potential public policy for mental patients. Am Psychol 37:349–359, 1982

12. Braun P, Kochansky G, Shapiro R, et al: Overview: deinstitutionalization of psychiatric patients, a critical review of outcome studies. Am J Psychiatry 138:736–749, 1981

13. Elpers JR, Crowell A: How many beds? An overview of resource planning. Hosp Community Psychiatry 33:755–761, 1982

14. Lamb HR: Structure: the neglected ingredient of community treatment. Arch Gen Psychiatry 37:1224–1228, 1980

15. Glick ID, Klar HM, Braff DL: Guidelines for hospitalization of chronic psychiatric patients. Hosp Community Psychiatry 35:934–936, 1984

16. Gunderson JG, Mosher LR: Psychotherapy of Schizophrenia. New York, J Aronson, 1975

17. Segal SP, Aviram U: The Mentally Ill in Community-Based Sheltered Care. New York, Wiley, 1978

18. May PRA: Schizophrenia: an overview of treatment methods, in Comprehensive Textbook of Psychiatry II. Edited by Freedman A, Kaplan HI, Sadock BJ. Baltimore, Williams & Wilkins, 1975

19. Ciompi L: Catamnestic long term study on the course of life and aging of schizophrenics. Schizophr Bull 6:606–618, 1980

20. Bleuler ME: On schizophrenic psychoses. Am J Psychiatry 136:1403–1409, 1979

21. Huber G, Gross G, Schuttler R, et al: Longitudinal studies of schizophrenic patients. Schizophr Bull 6:592–605, 1980

22. Harding C, Strauss JM: Unpublished paper presented at the Annual Meeting of the American Psychiatric Association. New York, NY, 1983

23. Herz M: Recognizing and preventing relapse in patients with schizophrenia. Hosp Community Psychiatry 35:344–349, 1984

24. Carpenter WT, Stephens JH, Rey AC: Early intervention vs continuous pharmacotherapy of schizophrenia. Psychopharmacol Bull 18:21–23, 1982

25. Anderson CM, Hogarty GE, Reiss DJ: Family treatment of adult schizophrenic patients: a psychoeducational approach. Schizophr Bull 6:490–505, 1980

26. Faloon RH, Boyd JL, McGill CW, et al: Family Management Training in the Community Care of Schizophrenia. New Directions for Mental Health Services, no. 12. San Francisco, Jossey-Bass, 1981, pp. 61–71

27. Vaughn CE, Leff JP: The influence of family and social factors on the course of psychiatric illness: a comparison of schizophrenic with depressed neurotic patients. Br J Psychiatry 129:123–137, 1976

28. Anthony WA, Cohen MR, Vitalo R: The measurement of rehabilitation outcome. Schizophr Bull 4:365–378, 1978

29. Strauss JS, Carpenter WT: The prognosis for schizophrenia: rationale for a multidimensional concept. Schizophr Bull 4:56, 1978

30. Anthony WA, Cohen MR, Vitalo R: The measurement of treatment outcome. Schizophr Bull 4:365–383, 1978

31. Weisbrod BA, Test MA, Stein LI: An alternative to mental hospital treatment. III. Economic benefit-cost analysis. Arch Gen Psychiatry 37:400–405, 1980

32. Murphy J, Datel W: A cost-benefit analysis of community versus institutional living. Hosp Community Psychiatry 27:165–170, 1976

33. Bachrach LL: Overview: model programs for chronic mental patients. Am J Psychiatry 137:1023–1031, 1980

34. Fenton FR, Tessier L, Struening EL: A comparative trial of home and hospital psychiatric care. Arch Gen Psychiatry 36:1073–1079, 1979

35. Talbott JA: Principles of successful programs for the chronic mentally ill. Unpublished paper

36. Hospital Association of New York State: Cost of Regulation Study. Albany, NY, Hospital Association of New York State, 1979

37. Blue Ribbon Commission on the Future of Public Inpatient Mental Health Services in Massachusetts: Mental Health Crossroads. Boston, Blue Ribbon Commission on the Future of Public Inpatient Mental Health Services in Massachusetts, 1981

38. Governor Carey's Health Advisory Council: Mental Health in the Year 2000. Albany, NY, Health Advisory Council, 1984

39. Stein LI, Ganser LJ: Wisconsin's system for funding mental health services, in Unified Mental Health Systems: Utopia Unrealized. Edited by Talbott JA. New Directions in Mental Health Services, no. 18. San Francisco, Jossey-Bass, 1983, pp. 25–32

CHAPTER 2

Recovery From Schizophrenia: A Personal Odyssey

MARCIA LOVEJOY

The author, who was diagnosed as having chronic process schizophrenia, describes her experiences as a patient in the treatment world of the chronic mentally ill, beginning at age 17. Over the next six years she was seen by four psychiatrists, was hospitalized eight times, attended day hospitals, lived in a foster care home, and received shock treatments, megavitamin therapy, and a variety of neuroleptic and antidepressant drugs. Eventually she developed a drinking problem and was forced to enter a chemical dependency treatment program. The first of many turning points in her illness came when a psychiatrist associated with the program believed she could recover and persuaded staff to work with her. The author defines hope as an essential element in the recovery process and emphasizes the importance of instilling hope for recovery in physicians, patients, and patient care staff. She attributes her recovery to multiple, sometimes nontraditional, treatment approaches and to the coping techniques she learned with the help of others.

Despite the many years I have spent being ill, I have grown and recovered from what many people believe is an incurable disease—chronic process schizophrenia. It is a label that can lead trained minds to slam shut and

This chapter first appeared in *Hospital and Community Psychiatry*, Volume 32, pp 809–812, 1984. Reprinted with permission.

to hopelessness and helplessness for the patient and his family. That label also carries no understanding or compassion to the general public of the suffering endured by patients with this problem.

When I formally entered the world of psychiatry in 1965, at age 17, doctors interviewed my family to verify that I had indeed been a strange and troubled child from a very young age. Two years later one doctor, who spent the most time researching my past, declared that I had been autistic since I was two. That label only hung a pall of failure over my family, who had always suspected something was wrong but never gave up hope that I would somehow outgrow it.

But my problems became bigger instead of smaller. The terrifying voices, sights, and smells that my parents had hoped were an overactive imagination were now labeled hallucinations. The medications that were vigorously administered only partially relieved the hallucinations. The sadly unemotional expression my face carried through all occasions, no matter how gay, now was labeled flat affect, and the medication seemed to only deepen that affect. I did have bursts of emotion, but always out of proportion to what others deemed normal. My mother said I was sensitive; the doctors said I had inappropriate outbursts. I distrusted most people out of fear of being hurt or rejected and often heard others laugh or put me down; that, of course, was labeled paranoia.

One day in deep curiosity I quickly read my hospital chart, left in my room by a careless intern. It was then that I became aware of the words that labeled me. At first I felt relieved. I thought, "Good, they know what is wrong with me; soon they will fix it for once and all and end my torment." I was influenced by television doctor shows in which brilliant minds quickly ended people's suffering. I patiently took my medication and waited for magic. It never came.

After almost a year, I started to look up those words in the library. Over several months I read hundreds of volumes; theories upon theories, book upon book postulated the basis for identifying symptoms, but not a single volume discussed cure. Very few even discussed ways of relieving the symptoms, and most ways seemed to center on pharmacologic research. The cause of my illness seemed to exist only on the future lab tables of research geneticists. Nothing made my present life better. I could find comfort only in Clifford Beers' book, *A Mind That Found Itself* (1), which seemed to outline his suffering only in a distant past. But one book in 100 years does not give one a lot of hope. The great lack of other books by recovered patients made me feel dismal. I wanted a ladder out of the morass of my problems, but what I read served to only light the morass, to clearly show me how hopeless it truly was.

CHRONIC TREATMENT

Meanwhile I entered the treatment world of a chronic mentally ill person. Chronic treatment is the lot of a person labeled chronically ill. The people working with me had no hope for my recovery; I met quite a few—a mixed bag of doctors, nurses, aides, recreation and occupational therapy personnel—as I drifted from hospitalizations to day programs to socialization groups, and so forth. In six years of treatment I would be seen by four psychiatrists, be hospitalized in two states a total of eight times, go to different day hospitals, receive shock treatments, live in a foster-care home, and receive megavitamins and three different neuroleptics (sometimes thousands of milligrams at a time, sometimes concurrently with three different antidepressants).

I was advised to avoid stress and to report an increase in symptoms. I was also told to smile more, but the few times I could bring myself to laugh at anything, I was told my laughter was inappropriate.

Periodically I saw patients physically and mentally abused by mental health workers who seemed sicker than we were. I saw many adults treated as children, never allowed to be angry or cry for even the most understandable reasons. I did not suffer physical abuse; I sat downcast on the hospital couches and waited patiently to be told to do or not do something. Meanwhile I either listened to voices or wished I were dead. Sometimes I believed I was dead, but mostly I just wished for death and sought relief in sleep, as did the rest of the chronic patients. Hundreds of times I gave up hope of ever finding help for my symptoms. I learned to watch my emotions and fear them and became obsessive about taking all medication as prescribed. It seemed over those years that the staff were as vigilant and fearful of my emotions as I was, or possibly I learned it from them; it is difficult to say.

Once early in my hospital years, staff decided that I should express my anger by pounding a punching dummy. I remember fearing that my emotions would become out of control as they had during my childhood. The numerous staff members present said they would prevent that loss of control and I could feel free to emote on the punching dummy. The last thing I remember of that event is the room looking strange. I later learned, when I awoke in the locked ward, that I had run amok and badly injured several staff. I was never charged with a crime, but as I went from program to program I lived out a sentence from that event: staff feared me. Often when I did not appear apathetic and dull, staff medicated me so they felt safer. I felt the shame and the guilt of an unpunished child.

In 1971 I experienced what has been labeled a psychotic exacerbation.

To me it meant I was sicker than usual. I remember speaking and no one hearing or listening to me. It never dawned on me that I was only thinking the words and no one but I could hear them. I was in a day hospital my mother had found that would take me for free if I lived in the area. My family had run out of hospitalization insurance and, despite my obvious need for the hospital, they could afford only this day program and a dear kindly lady who would see that I got there regularly.

One day in the three-month day program, that endless silence ended as suddenly as it began. I finished out the last half of the program a happy participant in group therapy, my first such involvement in six years. Before I had been allowed to attend only behavior or social groups and occupational or recreational therapy, for in those years chronic patients had not been considered good candidates for talk therapy.

ALCOHOL DEPENDENCY

When the program ended I was far from ready to get a job; I tried and failed miserably. In 1972 I went again to the same day hospital but became bored with the routine. I gave up on recovery and decided the less I felt, the better. I began to drink; it calmed my anxiety better than medication and helped numb my feelings just as the medication had. When the staff at the day hospital discovered my use of alcohol, they coerced me into a drug and alcohol treatment program. The psychiatrist who saw me in the hospital talked with me at length and then said something I will long remember. He said he had never seen anyone who was as sick as I who could express her symptoms as well as I could. He said he did not want to believe I could not recover, and, over the protestations of the chemical dependency folks, he insisted I learn their treatment approaches. This was a major turning point for me.

In that three-week chemical dependency program I learned that I had both a drinking and a psychiatric problem. The chemical dependency staff taught me specific "tools" to identify those behaviors, thoughts, and attitudes that triggered drinking and strategies for overcoming them. I learned to identify problems, to face them honestly, to examine all patterns of reaction and their results, to create new attitudes and approaches to deal with problems, to take responsibility for my life, and to make choices rather than simply being treated. I was empowered to change my life through the help of others rather than being a passive victim, and to replace self-pity and helplessness with courage and honesty.

However, the staff did not know how to teach me to identify those psychiatric stumbling blocks—attitudes, beliefs, situations, and conditions—that triggered emotional anguish for me. They convinced me that

I must find these triggers and develop my own tools with the aid of my psychiatrist and outpatient group therapy.

The staff of the chemical dependency program did help me to change a lot of attitudes, to trust, to have hope, and to gain more self-esteem. I never felt so much better; in fact, I secretly hoped that I was only an alcoholic and that this psychiatric stuff was a thing of the past. I left the hospital and went only to Alcoholics Anonymous because I preferred to be a recovered alcoholic rather than a mental patient, although I had received many warnings from program staff to treat both problems.

The emotional torment from the past quickly overwhelmed me, and I went back to the hospital, my psychiatrist, and my medication. However, I learned a valuable lesson and resumed searching, now with the aid of my psychiatrist and a supportive therapy group, for tools to identify the mysterious triggers to my emotional anguish and for the controls I could use to quell them.

I am still on this quest, although I now have a great deal of health. I have found many ways of handling symptoms so that my life is no longer out of control. I have come a long hard way. Many mental health professionals can say I was mislabeled and dismiss what I have experienced and learned; others can give me new labels. However, I hope some will not close their minds to what I have to offer. If the thousands of recovered people I have met these past six years mean anything, there is much to be learned from those who have been there and back.

PROGRESSION OF THE ILLNESS

I have learned a lot about my illness. I did not learn through a lone bit of genius but over time through experiencing the hell over and over, each time with more insight gained through the help of other people and my own self-examination.

My symptoms return in a series of stages, each with a corresponding physical and emotive component. The first stage is the most important; if I do not take appropriate steps to gain control here, each successive stage is more difficult.

In the first stage, I feel just a bit estranged from myself. From my eyes the world seems brighter and more sharply defined, and my voice seems to echo a bit. I start to feel uncomfortable being around people, and also uncomfortable in sharing my changing feelings.

In the second stage, everything appears a bit clouded. This cloudiness increases, as does my confusion and fear, especially fear of letting others know what is happening to me. I try to make logical excuses and to get control over the details of my life, and often make frantic efforts to organize everything; cleaning, cataloging, and self-involved activities are high. Songs on the radio begin to have greater meaning, and people seem to be looking at me strangely and laughing, giving me subtle messages I cannot understand. I start to misinterpret people's actions toward me, which increases my fear of losing control.

In the third stage, I believe I am beginning to understand why terrible things are happening to me: others are the cause of it. This belief comes with a clearing of sight, an increasing level of sound, and an increasing sensitivity to the looks of others. I carry on an argument with myself as to whether these things are true: "Is the FBI or the devil causing this? . . . No, that's crazy thinking. I wonder why people are making me crazy."

In the fourth and last stage, I become chaotic and see, hear, and believe all manner of things. I no longer question my beliefs, but act on them.

GUARDING AGAINST SYMPTOMS

Symptoms leave me in the same order they came. I have spent years at various stages, but now I spend a few days at most and experience only the first three stages. The first stage can appear easily, after I become overly tired or have been exposed to large groups of demanding folks with whom I feel uncomfortable. I have learned to watch for this stage and then to examine my recent environment. Getting more sleep, in conjunction with some quiet, and a low-sugar diet seem to aid in restoring the peace.

Sometimes I go into the second stage, which can easily scare me. The fear alone exacerbates my condition into the third stage. Physical illness can trigger many miserable days at this level of existence. In all stages, but especially this stage, keeping calm is important. It is very important that I talk to others, people who have helped in earlier crises and can remind me of things I can do to regain control. Sometimes it really helps for people just to acknowledge that I am feeling uncomfortable, and even though they believe it will pass they have empathy for what I am feeling; they do not try to argue me out of my feelings but comfort and guide me.

The psychiatrist who saw me in 1972 and had hope for me has been a powerful aid in the second stage. He has gone over my hospitalization records and found that 40 percent of the time I came in with a previously undiagnosed physical ailment such as pneumonia, cystitis, or anemia. When these conditions cleared up, so did my psychiatric problems.

Based on this finding, he later asked me to take my temperature the next time I hallucinated. At first I thought he was kidding, but I followed his orders and did find a correlation between raised temperature and psychotic symptoms. Taking my temperature became an important tool in my life, as did keeping a journal, which helped me feel less out of control in the second stage. I later learned to write and then repeat to myself positive statements, which helped dissolve the depreciating and frightening voices. Physical exercise became another tool to help me cope.

In 1975 I entered a halfway house with a special staff, one that had worked with a lot of ill people and, most important, knew how to have hope. Some of the staff were themselves recovered mentally ill people. Their very existence was a turning point of hope for me. The staff helped me continue to relearn to keep my attitude open and trusting toward people; even when I felt great distrust, they taught me to talk about my feelings and to find ways to believe in people. Their proposition was two-sided: I would work to become more open; they would work to become worthy of my trust. The fact that many of them spoke of recovery in the first person weighed heavily in my decision to trust. Although they failed at times, I learned to talk about even this most painful event and thus see it through to a good resolution.

The staff had developed a model program of peer group pressure and support. I met others who not only talked about the stages of symptoms but were actually gaining more understanding and control. Half the power of a symptom is relieved by understanding its cause and how to avoid having it become worse.

I learned that a way of judging the invalidity of a hallucination is to examine whether your surroundings appear different. If they do, there is a good chance that the voice, sight, and so forth is not real. I learned warming and relaxing techniques with my feet and legs ("grounding" techniques from bioenergetics); they relieved the power of my halluci-nations and could often end that estranged, disembodied feeling. What power and joy it was to feel relief and to have something with which to attack these terrible monsters of my soul! I began hatha-yoga techniques and felt better as my body became stronger. I was hypoglycemic and found a high-protein, low-carbohydrate diet greatly relieved my mood swings and gave me greater energy.

Attitude was the greatest struggle and, in the long run, I believe the most important. When I waited for a miracle drug or a magic therapy, I did not change—I stagnated. When I believed there was no hope for me, I found no avenues of change. When I distrusted all and feared being hurt, I acted unlovable and was disliked or at best ignored by others. Giving up distrust was the focus of my effort for many, many years. My counselor at the halfway house, a social worker at a support agency, and my psychiatrist talked to me about my distrust. They also talked to me about my spiritual relationship with God as I understand God to be.

Earlier physicians and treatment programs had ignored spirituality, but I believe it was important in my recovery.

THE IMPORTANCE OF HOPE

I wanted to have hope, and I wanted to believe I could live a life in control of my problems. I experienced a remarkable turning point at the halfway house. There I had met people who were truly recovered, some of whom were now even working as staff. You cannot imagine the kind of hope one gets from seeing, talking to, and hearing from other persons who know what you are going through because they have been there.

This hope gives one courage to change, to try, and to trust—all essential elements in recovery. Surgeons would rather not operate on a patient who feels no hope of recovery because they know that the patient's attitude is more powerful than anything they can do. In too many situations today neither psychiatrists nor their patients have any hope; the result is chronicity and endless suffering. I have found many people who have used all sorts of therapies to gain control or even eliminate symptoms, but all talk of how important it was to begin to have hope and take some action in their lives.

Psychiatry treats many people and gives them common labels. Some people have never been truly ill, but rather misunderstood. They are angry. Many arm themselves with lawyers and organize protests against psychiatry. They are shouting because they feel their voices are not being heard. Dozens of these groups around the world are learning to use the legal system to be heard. Their actions affect all of our lives and increasingly psychiatrists' practices. I do not believe, as Szasz does (2), that all psychiatrists are mistaken. I believe real problems exist for some of the patients treated by psychiatry.

However, I believe the treatment system is woefully inadequate and does not begin to address the need for hopeful and happy lives for those it purports to treat. I see psychiatrists who are busy pushing this theory of treatment over that theory of treatment—an egotistic waste of time. Every form of therapy has some merit with some patients, but the majority of clinical practices utilize only one or two approaches and do not serve 80 percent of the patients. I have hope that the practice of psychiatry can change. A psychiatrist believed in me when I did not believe in myself and used multiple approaches in addressing my problems. He sought the answers *with* me rather than *for* me. There are also several other mental health professionals to whom I am indebted.

In my travels I have met many discouraged physicians numbly living out their hopeless lives, which is reflected in the quality of care they provide their patients. This hopeless attitude pervades their work, their staff, and, finally, their patients. This situation should not exist and I hope it can be changed.

When asked by the staff of the TV news show *Nightline* if I would mind being introduced in an interview as a schizophrenic, I told them yes, I would mind, that I was not a practicing schizophrenic. I meant that at this time my life is not out of control and I practice health, and health is a continuum. For me it takes effort, although on most days very little effort. I now have hope and knowledge—a combination that ensures my health and is the bedrock of recovery and relief from suffering. I used to be ashamed of being mentally ill. I am not ashamed anymore.

REFERENCES

1. Beers CW: A Mind That Found Itself: An Autobiography, 5th ed. New York, Longmans, Green, 1921
2. Szasz TS: The Myth of Mental Illness: Foundations of a Theory of Personal Conduct, rev. ed. New York, Harper and Row, 1974

CHAPTER 3

Epidemiology of Chronic Mental Disorder

HOWARD H. GOLDMAN, M.D., PH.D.
RONALD W. MANDERSCHEID, PH.D.

Five years ago, the problem of the chronic mental patient was an emerging issue in mental health policy. The American Psychiatric Association's publication, *The Chronic Mental Patient* (1), was one of several important documents that addressed concern for the mentally disabled (2–4). It provided a comprehensive overview of data, service concepts, models, plans, and programs relating to the chronic mentally ill, including an excellent chapter on the scope of the problem by Minkoff (5).

Since publication of *The Chronic Mental Patient*, additional work related to the epidemiology of chronic mental disorder has been completed. Notably, the document *Toward a National Plan for the Chronically Mental Ill (NPCMI)* (6), based on recommendations and data presented by the President's Commission on Mental Health (PCMH) (4), developed a definition of the target population and provided an unduplicated count of the chronic mentally ill (7). This chapter reviews studies in the epidemiology of chronic mental disorder published after 1978 that are national in scope or that inform the process of delimiting, defining, locating, counting, and characterizing the chronic mentally ill. This work follows the conceptual and organizational framework developed for *NPCMI*, bor-

Portions of this chapter first appeared in Goldman et al: Defining and counting the chronically mentally ill. Hosp Community Psychiatry 32:22–27, 1981; and in Talbott J (Ed): The Chronic Mental Patient: Five Years Later. Orlando, FL, Grune & Stratton, 1984. Reprinted with permission.

rowing text and supplementing it with new findings and new approaches to defining and counting the chronically mentally ill. The data that guided the estimates presented in *NPCMI* (6) are already quite old. Community estimates were based on 1973 data and institutional estimates were based on 1977 data. They are, however, the only data available for providing an *unduplicated* count of the population at about the same point in time. New data are becoming available and new issues are emerging, such as chronic mentally ill children and youth, homelessness, the "new chronic patient," and incarceration of chronically mentally ill persons. This paper provides an update on the epidemiology of chronic mental disorder. It points a direction for future research and for a new project to redefine and recount the chronically mentally ill.

WHO ARE THE CHRONIC MENTALLY ILL?

Sylvia Frumkin is chronically mentally ill (8); so are Jim Logue and the Duck Lady from Don Drake's "The Forsaken" (9). Al, Luther, Agnes, Morning Star, and Angelita are five patients who introduce *NPCMI* (6). The Box Lady and her tragic death is the subject of a report in *The New York Times* (10). They are all chronically mentally ill, as are more than two million others we label by this broad term. The term "chronic mentally ill" presents several problems: It has been difficult to define operationally. It stigmatizes individuals with connotations of hopelessness and inevitable deterioration. And it obscures the heterogeneity of the population, grouping together a diversity of individuals under a single pessimistic rubric that some fear becoming a self-fulfilling prophecy (1, 6, 11, 12). In spite of these limitations, we continue to use the term because of its widespread acceptance.

Prior to the era of deinstitutionalization, the chronic mentally ill were easier to identify and count; they were the long-term residents of psychiatric hospitals. Today, these institutions are no longer home to the majority of persons disabled by chronic mental illness. One consequence of the shifts in the pattern and locus of mental health care arising from deinstitutionalization is a lack of definitive information on the scope of the problem of chronic mental illness. Sources of data, like the affected individuals and their services, have been dispersed and decentralized. The difficulty is compounded by the absence of consensus on a definition that would delimit the target population.

Broadly speaking, a chronic condition is characterized by a long duration of illness, which may include periods of seeming wellness interrupted by flare-ups of acute symptoms, and secondary disabilities. This simple characterization is applicable to chronic mental illness, but the task of identifying persons who are chronically mentally ill is not at all straightforward. Although it is true that most such persons "are, have been, or might have been, but for the deinstitutionalization movement, on the rolls of long-term mental institutions, especially State hospitals" (13), any attempt to specify the attributes of state hospital patients must take into account the dynamic nature of clinical judgments about these patients.

Perceptions about the appropriateness of patient placement in state hospitals and other psychiatric facilities have been changing rapidly in recent years (14), and there is every reason to think they will continue to change in the future. As knowledge about the heterogeniety of patients' needs increases, the formulation of appropriateness should evolve (15). As the number and variety of community-based services expand, however, clinical judgments about appropriateness change. This variability in the assessment of needs is to be expected and encouraged in a dynamic service system.

DELIMITING THE TARGET POPULATION

Assessing the prevalence of chronic mental illness is complicated by the dynamic, episodic course of severe mental disorders. Von Korff and Parker (16), who propose several models for determining the prevalence of chronic episodic disease, conclude: "The prevalence of episodic disease is not solely a function of incidence and duration. . . . [It] is a function of incidence, average episode duration, and average number of episodes" (p 84). Some individuals recover; some have histories marked by exacerbations and remissions; others have a persistent, deteriorating course.

Chronic mental illness encompasses more than episodic disorder; it implies impairment and disability that are based upon community reaction. Minkoff's attempt (5) to define and count the chronic mentally ill distinguished persons who are severely *mentally ill* (defined by diagnosis), those who are *mentally disabled* (defined by level of disability), and those who are *chronic mental patients* (defined by duration of hospitalization).

These three dimensions—diagnosis, disability, duration—are sufficiently operationalizable to serve as criteria for delimiting the target population (see Figure 1). We can begin with the following general description: The chronic mentally ill population suffers from emotional disorders that interfere with their functional capacities in relation to such primary aspects of daily life as self-care, interpersonal relationships, and work or schooling, and that may often necessitate prolonged mental health care.

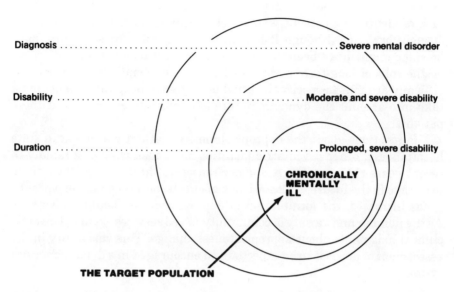

Diagnosis .... Severe mental disorder

Disability .... Moderate and severe disability

Duration .... Prolonged, severe disability

CHRONICALLY
MENTALLY
ILL

THE TARGET POPULATION

Figure 1.   The Dimensions of Chronic Mental Illness: Diagnosis, Disability, Duration. Adapted from the *National Plan for the Chronically Mentally Ill.*

Diagnosis

There is general agreement that psychoses and other major disorders predominate among this population; that is, organic mental disorders, schizophrenic disorders, major affective disorders, paranoid disorders, and other psychotic disorders (17). Other disorders may also lead to chronic mental disability. Recently proposed changes in the "listings" of mental impairments for disability programs of the Social Security Administration also include the anxiety disorders, somatoform disorders, and personality disorders. Furthermore, alcohol and drug abuse disorders and mental retardation may complicate the course of severe mental disorders (occasionally becoming designated as the primary diagnosis) or may become chronically disabling conditions themselves. Among children, schizophrenia, childhood autism, and some behavior disorders may lead to chronic disability; the same may be said of nonpsychotic organic mental disorders, or "senility without psychosis" (as designated in the *International Classification of Diseases*: 8th Edition [18]), among the elderly.[1]

---

[1]This was the classification of diseases used in the 1977 National Nursing Home Survey that reported data on "senility without psychosis."

Disability

Most definitions of disability center on the concept of functional incapacity; for example, "partial or total impairment of instrumental (usually vocational or homemaking) role performance" (5). One statutory definition refers to a condition that "results in substantial functional limitations in three or more of the following areas of major life activity: (i) self-care, (ii) receptive and expressive language, (iii) learning, (iv) mobility, (v) self-sufficiency" (Public Law 95-602) (19). However, objective measures of these "functional limitations" are not now in widespread use, although progress is being made in measurement methodologies (20, 21).

Chronicity of disability may be operationally defined by Social Security Disability Insurance (SSDI) and Supplemental Security Income (SSI) eligibility in terms of receipt of SSDI or SSI payments. Eligibility implies that the beneficiary has been unable to "engage in any substantial gainful activity" because of a disorder "which has lasted or can be expected to last for a continuous period of not less than 12 months." General agreement exists that approval of SSI eligibility is a measure of chronic disability for noninstitutionalized persons. Similar vocational criteria are common to other definitions of disability, such as those used in the Survey of Disabled Adults (Social Security Administration) and the Survey of Income and Education (U.S. Bureau of the Census). Chronicity also may be inferred from the need for extended hospitalization or other forms of supervised residence or sheltered work.

Duration

To infer disability from the need for extended hospitalization or supervised residential care requires specifying some duration of residence. Most would agree that one year of continuous institutionalization in a state mental hospital or of residence in a nursing home would qualify as a measure of chronic mental disability. However, at least half of the chronic mentally ill population are not continuously institutionalized (see Figure 2). Although these latter individuals reside in the community, many of them were hospitalized in the past or are hospitalized during the course of the year. Some formula is necessary for determining what duration of hospitalization to use as a criterion for chronicity for the chronic mentally ill living in the community.

Treated prevalence estimates may be obtained by reference to the National Reporting Program of the National Institute of Mental Health (NIMH), Division of Biometry and Epidemiology, which uses a three-month period of follow-up for providing data on extended hospitalization.

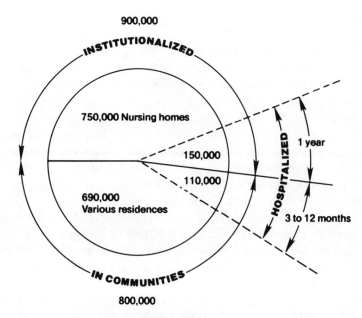

Figure 2. The Location of the Chronically Mentally Ill, United States, 1977. Adapted from the *National Plan for the Chronically Mentally Ill.*

Eighty percent of all patients admitted to private psychiatric hospitals and general hospital psychiatric units are discharged within 90 days (22, 23). Likelihood of release diminishes after this point; hence, we may consider that these unreleased patients represent an intermediate-stay (3–12 months) population of the chronic mentally ill (see Figure 2).

It should be noted that some persons with characteristics fitting the diagnosis and disability criteria have received short-term (less than 90 days) inpatient care, solely outpatient care from a medical or mental health professional, or no care at all save what their families or other natural support groups have provided. Although we are unable definitely to locate or enumerate such individuals, we include them in the target population. Prolonged functional disability caused or aggravated by severe mental disorders, not former hospitalization, is the chief distinguishing characteristic of chronic mental illness.

THE CHRONIC MENTALLY ILL

There have been several recent attempts to operationally define the chronic mentally ill. The definitions reviewed here were developed to provide estimates of the size of the population. They are not conceptual definitions; they are practical definitions designed to identify mentally disabled individuals who are eligible for services and to estimate the scope of the problem of chronic mental illness.

The Community Support Program (CSP) of NIMH developed the following parameters for eligibility for its target population of noninstitutionalized chronically mentally ill. "Severe mental disability [must satisfy at least one of the following]: A single episode of hospitalization in the last five years of at least six months duration; or two or more hospitalizations within a 12-month period" (24). This definition includes individuals with nonchronic conditions who may have required two brief hospitalizations in one year and excludes multiple-admission chronic patients who have been kept out of the hospital for 12 months. Furthermore, it is difficult to obtain national data estimates by using the CSP formula.

CSP continues to change its definition of program eligibility to ameliorate problems associated with earlier definitions. Recently, CSP has attempted to focus on assessing functional disabilities and to minimize reliance on a history of prior institutionalization. This opens eligibility to the mentally disabled who may not have been hospitalized due to current deinstitutionalization efforts. Unfortunately, preliminary field tests of the reliability of these new eligibility criteria were disappointing (25). Moreover, in a 1981 study sponsored by CSP, Macro Systems found that definitions of the chronic mentally ill vary from state to state.

CSP also sponsored a needs assessment project conducted by the Human Services Research Institute. This project developed a series of models for estimating the needs and size of the chronic mentally ill population in the community (26). The method relies on data that are easily obtained. Specifically, it relies on national and state counts of persons receiving SSI and SSDI for reason of mental illness, on sample counts of persons awarded SSI and SSDI benefits in recent years for reason of mental illness by zip code area, and on full or sample counts of chronic mentally ill persons in publicly funded community mental health programs by SSI and SSDI status. National data from this project will be discussed later.

Szymanski and colleagues (27) described three methods for estimating the local prevalence of the chronic mentally ill who might need CSPs. The first method identifies patients who require outpatient care and who were hospitalized in the past. The second method identifies patients who require rehospitalization during a specified period of time following a prior hospitalization. The third method identifies outpatients who have a diagnosis of schizophrenia. These approaches to estimating the size of the populations are all derived from treated prevalence data, which tend to underestimate true prevalence. However, such data are readily available at low cost for regional planning. Other methods for local needs assessment have been described by Warheit et al. (28) and, more recently, by Ashbaugh (29).

NPCMI (6) presents the following definition of the target population based on the dimensions of diagnosis, disability, and duration:

> The chronically mentally ill population encompasses persons who suffer certain mental or emotional disorders (organic brain syndrome, schizophrenia, recurrent depressive and manic-depressive disorders, paranoid and other psychoses, plus other disorders that may become chronic) that erode or prevent the development of their functional capacities in relation to (three or more of) such primary aspects of daily life as personal hygiene and self-care, self-direction, interpersonal relationships, social transactions, learning, and recreation, and that erode or prevent the development of their economic self-sufficiency. Most such individuals have required institutional care of extended duration, including intermediate-term hospitalization (90 days to one year in a single year), long-term hospitalization (one year or longer in the preceding five years), nursing home placement on account of a diagnosed mental condition or diagnosis of senility without psychosis. Some such individuals have required short-term hospitalization (less than 90 days), others have received treatment from a medical or mental health professional solely on an outpatient basis, or despite their needs, have received no treatment in the professional-care service system. Thus, included in the target population are persons who are or were formerly "residents" of institutions (public and private psychiatric hospitals and nursing homes), and persons who are at high risk of institutionalization because of persistent mental disability. (p. 2–11)

LOCATING THE POPULATION

Bearing in mind the caveat concerning the dynamic nature of any definition of this population, we propose to outline a series of separate segments of the population of the chronic mentally ill. The numbers of chronic mentally ill persons in each of these segments may be determined by several methods. Over time, these numbers are subject to change because of the movement of people from one location to another.

Institutional Residents

For the purposes of this report, the institutionalized chronic mentally ill are those individuals with any psychiatric diagnosis in mental hospitals for more than one year and those individuals in nursing homes (as defined by the National Center for Health Statistics) with a diagnosed mental condition or a diagnosis of senility without psychosis. The latter are included because simple senility, either alone or in a combination with other chronic medical conditions, was a reason for admission to a state mental hospital prior to policies encouraging deinstitutionalization and the transfer or diversion of the elderly into nursing homes.

Community Residents

Within communities, the chronic mentally ill are those individuals in a variety of residential settings (for example, with families, in boarding homes, in community residential facilities, in single occupancy hotel rooms, in the streets, or in correctional facilities) who are considered to be disabled by any one of several criteria (for example, SSI/SSDI eligibility, episodic or prolonged hospitalization, inability to work). This community-dwelling segment may be subdivided into several groups on the basis of their location, their utilization of mental health facilities, and the level and type of their disability.

COUNTING THE CHRONIC POPULATION

Having defined the target population in terms of disability and location, we now turn to determining their number. As Table 1 indicates, estimates of the number of the chronic mentally ill range from 1.7 million to 2.4 million, including 900,000 who are institutionalized. Table 2 presents estimates of the types of disabilities suffered by persons with chronic illness and their utilization of mental health facilities. These estimates of the total number of chronic mentally ill are derived from a number of sources, including true prevalence estimates of chronic mental disorders, community estimates of chronic mental disability, and treated prevalence data on chronic mental patients.

Chronic Mental Disorders—True Prevalence Estimates

The field of psychiatric epidemiology has expanded dramatically since the publication of the report of the President's Commission on Mental Health (4), *The Chronic Mental Patient* (1), and the other seminal work on the chronic mentally ill written in the late 1970s. Robins (30) and Weissman and Klerman (31) herald the advances of the field and their promise for reliable and valid community estimates of the incidence and prevalence of specific mental disorders. Currently, the NIMH Epidemiologic Catchment Program is sponsoring a five-site field study of the epidemiology of mental disorder in the United States. Data from this multisite study will be available in the near future to guide estimates of the prevalence of severe and chronic mental disorder.

Table 1. Estimates of the number of the chronic mentally ill, United States, 1975-1977

Institutionalized Population	
Location (unduplicated count)	
Mental health facilities[1]	150,000
Nursing homes[2]	
Residents with mental disorder[3]	300,000
Residents with mental and physical disorder	450,000
Subtotal	900,000
Community Population	
Level of disability (unduplicated count)	
Severe[4]	800,000
Moderate[5] and severe	1,500,000
Subtotal (range)	800,000 to 1,500,000
Total[6]	1,700,000 to 2,400,000

[1]Residents for one year or more in the following facility types: state and county hospitals, Veterans Administration inpatient facilities, private psychiatric hospitals, residential treatment centers, or community mental health centers (source of estimates: Division of Biometry and Epidemiology, NIMH, 1975).
[2]Universe of 1.3 million residents of skilled nursing and intermediate care facilities sampled by National Center for Health Statistics, National Nursing Home Survey, 1977.
[3]Residents with a primary diagnosis of 797 (senility without psychosis) or from section V of the *International Classification of Diseases*, 8th ed. (source: National Nursing Home Survey, 1977).
[4]Includes individuals with a mental disorder unable to work at all for one year and those who could work only occasionally or irregularly. (Source of estimates: Urban Institute, Comprehensive Service Needs Survey, 1973, and National Center for Health Statistics, Survey of Disabled Adults, 1966).
[5]Includes so-called "partially disabled" individuals whose work (including housework) was limited by a mental disorder (source of estimates: Urban Institute, Comprehensive Service Needs Survey, 1973).
[6]For purposes of *NPCMI*, the lower figure (1.7 million), representing the severely disabled chronic mentally ill, will be used as the size of the target population.

In the absence of such data, *NPCMI* relied on data estimates from PCMH (4), based largely on a review paper by Dohrenwend et al. (32). *NPCMI* also contained data reported in Minkoff's secondary analysis (5). This section will review the prevalence estimates developed for *NPCMI* and will mention some newer sources that would modify these estimates.

According to the President's Commission on Mental Health (4), there are approximately two million people in the United States who could be

Table 2. Estimates of the number of the chronic mentally ill by type of disability and use of mental health facilities (duplicated counts), United States, 1975–1977

Type of Disability	
Receiving SSI/SSDI[1]	550,000
Complete work disability[2]	350,000
Activity limitation[3]	700,000
Use of Mental Health Facilities[4]	
Admissions (length of stay ≥ 90 days)	150,000
Readmissions[5]	650,000

[1]Source: Anderson (47) cites the *Social Security Bulletin*, Volume 44, March 1981, pp 2–48.
[2]Prevalence of disability in 18- to 64-year-old population (44).
[3]Prevalence of disability in population three years or older (44).
[4]Facilities include state and county mental hospitals, private psychiatric hospitals, psychiatric units in general hospitals, and residential treatment centers (source: Division of Biometry and Epidemiology, NIMH, 1975).
[5]Readmission counts will overestimate chronic patients. Some patients with less severe disorders are admitted many times for brief admissions (source: Division of Biometry and Epidemiology, NIMH, 1975).

given a diagnosis of schizophrenia. Approximately 600,000 of them are in active treatment during a given year, accounting for more than 500,000 admissions in the specialty mental health sector. Any individual given a diagnosis of schizophrenia is at risk of becoming chronically mentally ill. However, because of the existence of other acute syndromes that mimic the overt symptoms of schizophrenia, but do not invariably become progressive or chronic (for example, schizophreniform psychosis, brief reactive psychosis), not all of the two million individuals are to be counted among the chronic mentally ill. Estimates of the number of chronic mentally ill individuals with a diagnosis of schizophrenia would range from 500,000 to 900,000. There is considerable controversy in the literature concerning the prevalence of schizophrenia. Researchers from Taylor and Abrams (33) to Pope and Lipinski (34) have been questioning reported rates of schizophrenia, asserting they are overestimates that confuse schizophrenia with psychotic manifestations of affective disorder. Carpenter et al. and Strauss (35, 36) have emphasized the difficulty in predicting chronicity from symptomatology in the schizophrenic disorders unless diagnostic criteria are based on duration of symptomatology. They assert that chronic deterioration is overestimated. Further, they find that only prior disability and chronicity accurately predict future disability and chronicity.

Serious depression has a prevalence rate ranging from 0.3 percent to 1.2 percent (4). Assuming that the lower end of the range represents the population at highest risk of chronicity, there are perhaps 600,000 to 800,000 chronically and severely depressed individuals in the United States. Since publication of the PCMH report (4), several reviews of the epidemiology of affective disorders have been published (37–39). However, none of these papers deals directly with the issue of severity or chronicity. Prien (40) reviews the data on the prevalence of chronic affective disorder, concluding that about 20 percent of individuals with affective disorders have a chronic course. However, not all such patients suffer persistent disabilities.

Psychosis in the elderly (primarily organic mental disorders, predominantly chronic) is estimated to account for between 600,000 to 1,250,000 individuals (4). These estimates are sustained by recent reviews of the epidemiology of senile dementia (41, 42). All authors stress the expected increases in this population as the large cohort born during the postwar baby boom survive into the senium. This aspect of chronic mental illness may be the single most critical problem for the future (43).

Other more prevalent disorders, such as personality disorders (7 percent prevalence), alcoholism and alcohol abuse (5 to 10 percent), and drug abuse and misuse (1 to 10 percent, depending on the type of drug) may become chronic or may be complicated by chronic mental disorder. However, only a small minority of these individuals are part of the target population (6).

Chronic Mental Disability—Community Estimates

Currently, there are four major sources of national data on chronic mental disability in the community: the U.S. Bureau of the Census (44) Survey of Income and Education done in 1976, the National Center for Health Statistics (45) Survey of Disabled Adults done in 1966 and reported in 1970, a 1973 Comprehensive Service Needs Study conducted by the Urban Institute (46) for the Department of Health, Education and Welfare, and a 1978 Social Security Administration Survey of Disability and Work (66). These studies indicate that there are between 350,000 and 800,000 individuals severely disabled by emotional disorder in the community and perhaps an additional 700,000 people with moderate disability.

According to data published by the U.S. Bureau of the Census, based on 1976 estimates of disability in the community, approximately 700,000 persons three years of age or older (2.5 percent of a total of 28 million disabled people) have an "activity limitation" due to severe mental disturbance. A total of 350,000 individuals between the ages of 18 and 64 have some work disability (including total disability) secondary to severe emotional disturbance (44).

Extrapolations from the Urban Institute study indicate that approximately 800,000 individuals in the community have a severe mental disability, and 700,000 more are moderately or partially disabled (46). These data are corroborated by the most recent Social Security Administration survey, which estimated that approximately 1.07 million adults between the ages of 20 and 64 living in households were disabled by emotional disorder (15). Figure 3 shows the distribution of the SSI/SSDI recipient population for 1978 and the magnitude of the chronically mentally ill within this population. Further estimates from the Social Security Administration suggest that 550,000 of the severely disabled are receiving Supplemental Security Income or Social Security Disability Insurance benefits (47).

Chronic Mental Patients—Treated Prevalence Data

Estimates of the number of chronic mental patients may also be derived from two sources of treated prevalence data. The first source is national data from the National Reporting Program of the NIMH Division of Biometry and Epidemiology, the Veterans Administration, and the Long-Term Care Statistics Branch of the National Center for Health Statistics. The second source is the Monroe County (New York) case register. Both data sources suggest that the number of chronic mental patients is approximately 1.7 million.

The Monroe County figure is derived (by Carl Taube of the NIMH Division of Biometry and Epidemiology) through extrapolation from the 10-year follow-up experience of a cohort of state mental hospital patients from Rochester State Hospital in 1962. Although generalization from these data is problematic, this estimate provides a useful verification of the estimates derived from the national data.

The national data from 1977 (66) provide the following estimates: the institutional population totals about 900,000 and includes two major subdivisions of chronic mental patients based on place of residence: specialty mental health sector facilities and nursing homes. Approximately 150,000 chronic mental patients are inpatients in the specialty mental health sector. Based on a 1973 study of resident patients in an unrepresentative sample of state mental hospitals in 13 states (and confirmed by a 1979 survey of a representative sample), an estimated 60 percent of the resident census had been in continuous residence for one year or more. Applying this estimate to the current (1977) resident census of 160,000 patients in state and county mental hospitals, we can conclude that there

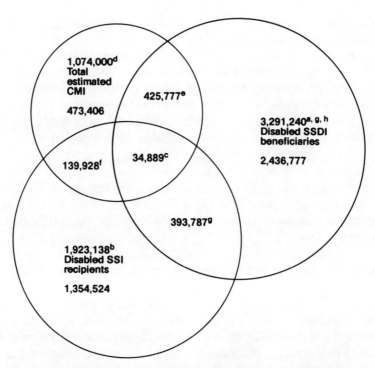

Figure 3. Preliminary Estimates of Chronically Mentally Ill Persons Receiving SSI and SSDI Payments as of December 31, 1978.

[a]Annual Statistical Supplement, 1977–79. Social Security Bulletin, 1978. (table 120).

[b]Program and Demographic Characteristics of Supplemental Security Beneficiaries, 1978. SSA Pub. No. 13:11977, April 1980. (table 4).

[c]Based on two samples of successful, noninstitutionalized, adult (18–64) applicants (SSDI—8,068; SSI—4,184) in 1975–77.

[d]Estimated from Survey of Disability and Work, 1978.

[e]Estimate derived from items c and d.

[f/g]Program and Demographic Characteristics of Supplemental Security Beneficiaries, 1978. SSA Pub. No. 13:11977, April 1980. (table 1).

[h]Includes 2,879,774 disabled workers; 282,782 disabled adult children and spouses; and 128,684 disabled widows.

are approximately 100,000 chronic mental patients institutionalized in these facilities. An additional 50,000 (crude estimate) are long-term (more than one year) residents of other specialty facilities. Approximately 20,000 are in other facilities, including private psychiatric hospitals and CMHC inpatient units.

There were an estimated 750,000 chronic mental patients in nursing homes out of a total resident population of 1.3 million in 1977. This figure, which may be a slight overestimate, encompasses two groups of individuals: those with a primary mental disorder including mental retardation and senility (approximately 300,000) and those with a physical disorder and a mental disorder, especially senility without psychosis (approximately 450,000). The second group represents a population of elderly individuals who probably would have been admitted to the state mental hospitals in the pre-deinstitutionalization era. For this reason, both subpopulations of nursing home residents are considered chronic mental patients (48).

Data on prior care in a state mental hospital indicate that in 1977 perhaps only 100,000 nursing home residents were transferred directly from a state mental hospital. Although this number strikes many as low, several explanations are possible—underreporting, successful diversion programs barring the elderly from public long term care hospitals in recent years, and transfers from other nursing homes rather than directly from state and county mental hospitals. Data suggest that nursing homes may indeed be the new "back wards in the community" (49).

The *community population* of chronic mental patients with severe disability numbers approximately 800,000. An additional 700,000 individuals have a partial disability due to a mental condition. The patterns of service utilization by this population are more difficult to estimate because the individuals in the population are more dynamic, possibly using several facilities during the course of a year. They are also more mobile, living in a wide variety of residential treatment settings—for example, with their families, in congregate care, in residences with single room occupancy, in board and care homes, in the streets, or in correctional facilities. Using treated prevalence data alone will represent an undercount of the community population, some of whom receive no treatment or receive care exclusively in other sectors, such as the general health care, social welfare, or criminal justice systems.

The severely disabled community population may be divided into two subgroups on the basis of utilization of specialty mental health services. The first is the intermediate-length-of-stay hospitalized population composed of approximately 110,000 individuals who remained in the hospital for a period between 3 and 12 months following admission to state and county mental hospitals (about 80,000), private psychiatric hospitals (about 10,000), residential treatment centers (about 15,000), and general hospital psychiatric units (about 5,000).

The second severely disabled community group is the ambulatory population of approximately 700,000 chronic mental patients. The estimates of the service utilization of this ambulatory population are less reliable than the other estimates. Of these chronic patients, at least 200,000 are readmissions to state and county mental hospitals for brief (less than 90 days) hospitalization, another estimated 100,000 are chronic patients in community mental health centers, and the balance are chronic patients being cared for in other specialty facilities in the community. The 700,000 figure represents a very conservative estimate, since it is based on treated prevalence data and therefore does not account for the chronic ambulatory population in other sectors, such as primary care and social welfare, or the number of untreated individuals, including the homeless chronic mentally ill.

Criticism of the role of community mental health centers in the care of chronic patients (2, 50, 51) has led to several studies of the prevalence of patients with severe and chronic disorder in such facilities (25, 52). Abt Associates, under contract to NIMH, is examining this issue in detail. Unpublished preliminary data indicate that community mental health centers continue to see a significant number of chronic patients even if this is not their primary target population. As Langsley (53) reminds us, we need more than biometric data to answer the critical question: "Do community mental health centers treat patients?"

Data on the quality and appropriateness of services are limited. However, data on service utilization are plentiful. We do know that in 1975 there were approximately 650,000 patient readmissions to state and county mental hospitals, private psychiatric hospitals, and psychiatric units in general hospitals. All of these readmitted patients are not chronic mental patients; however, they may be counted among the 800,000 to 1,500,000 individuals moderately and severely disabled by mental disorder who spend most of the year in the community.

These chronic mental patients live in a variety of community residences. A service delivery assessment in Health and Human Services region III estimated that between 300,000 and 400,000 of these chronic mental patients reside in community residential facilities, such as board and care homes (54). These domiciliary care residences and single-room-occupancy hotels often are criticized as substandard, isolating, and a form of "transinstitutionalization" and continued neglect (1, 49, 54).

However, not all chronic patients are transinstitutionalized. Some return to their families. Although approximately 65 percent of discharged mental patients return home (55, 56), not all of these are chronic. Several studies report that approximately one in four chronic patients is discharged to his or her family (5). The analysis of data from the Social Security Administration's 1978 Survey of Disability and Work indicates that 59 percent of the 1.07 million mentally disabled Americans living in households were married and residing with a spouse (15).

Emerging Issues

There are three emerging problems that deserve comment with respect to the chronic mentally ill population, although few data are currently available to address them. These are the problems of chronic mentally ill children and adolescents, the young adult chronic patient, and the homeless chronic mentally ill.

The child mental health field traditionally has hesitated to label young people as "chronic," preferring instead to focus on prevention and correction of problems in psychosocial development. However, the field recognizes the long-term care and treatment needs of a population estimated at 70,000 children and youth in the United States (6). That population has been defined in *NPCMI* (6) as individuals under the age of 18 with a mental disorder, such as autism and other pervasive developmental disorders, childhood schizophrenia, and severe behavior disorder, that produces emotional and/or organic impairment of at least one year's duration characterized by functional limitations in self-care, perceptive and expressive language, learning, self-direction, and basic social skills. *NPCMI* further specified the need for a "combination and sequence of special, interdisciplinary or generic care, treatment, or other services . . . of extended duration" (6, p A-42).

Detailed epidemiologic data are lacking on mental disorders in children. The *NPCMI* estimate of 70,000 was based on NIMH data and included 50,000 children in hospital and other residential treatment settings and 20,000 nonhospitalized children and adolescents. These data remain the most complete estimates available to the field.

The young adult chronic patient has been described in the literature as more likely to have multiple problems, more likely to be transient, more difficult to treat, and less likely to have had continuous contact with the mental health care system (57–59). Although the rates of disorder may be no different in this age group (typically 18–35) compared to other age cohorts, the number of persons with chronic disorders is likely to be substantially larger because of the baby boom phenomenon between 1946 and 1964. NIMH data suggest that a segment of this population is replacing the elderly in state hospitals (60). Projections of current trends in this service setting anticipate an expansion of state hospitals in the future; this would revise the downward trend in resident population that has occurred since 1955 (61). Among the young adult chronic patients participating in the CSP, results showed that young chronics tend to receive nonpsychotic diagnoses, exhibit deviant and disruptive behaviors, and use mental health and other services at higher rates than do older chronic patients. Clinical histories varied by age group in expected ways, and demographic characteristics and degree of psychiatric disability tended to be similar across age groups (62). Development of effective services for this chronic population will be a major challenge of the coming decade.

The homeless chronically mentally ill represent an equal challenge. Estimates of the entire homeless population range from a daily count of 250,000 to 550,000 (Department of Housing and Urban Development) to an annual total of 2,500,000 (National Coalition for the Homeless). Based on a review of available local studies, one of us (R.W.M.) has found that deinstitutionalized chronic mentally ill persons appear to represent about 25 percent of the homeless population in urban areas. When combined with a second subgroup, chronically or acutely mentally ill persons who have been diverted from inpatient care or who have rejected psychiatric treatment, the mentally ill appear to constitute from 40 to 60 percent of the homeless population in urban areas. These estimates may be conservative, since most local studies are based on shelter users, and the mentally ill are less likely to use shelters. Thus, the number of chronic mentally ill individuals who are homeless cannot be clearly specified at the present time. However, estimated most conservatively, the number would be considerable.

An ancillary problem is the use of correctional facilities by the mentally ill homeless. As with the homeless population, little factual information is available on the numbers of mentally ill persons in correctional facilities on a given day or during an entire year. The National Coalition for Jail Reform has estimated that approximately 700,000 incarcerations of mentally ill persons occur each year in local and county jails. Granted the heavy representation of chronic mentally ill persons in the homeless population, it is reasonable to assume that they are also represented among the mentally ill incarcerated in correctional settings.

THE CHALLENGE FOR THE FUTURE

The technical criteria for defining the chronic mentally ill described in this chapter establish the objective boundaries of the target population, which are vital to the activities of planners and policymakers. But they do no more than hint at the clinical, socioeconomic, ethnic, and cultural heterogeneity of this population. Data from several national surveys are currently being analyzed, and a few reports on the characteristics of chronic patients in national programs have been published (63–65). But data cannot convey any sense of the individual people referred to, their frailties and strengths, their suffering and that of their families, their hope and striving, however faltering, for normalcy.

The chronic mentally ill population includes persons whose clinical conditions and functional disabilities vary widely at any point in time and, moreover, change over time. Kramer's projections for the year 2005 indicate that chronic mental disability will increase dramatically (43). Variability makes an accurate determination of the size and nature of the population extremely difficult. At best, we can provide an estimate to guide national policymakers in a more scientific assessment of needs. Currently, we are beginning to update the data reported above. The limiting factor in this endeavor is the availability of data for a single year on both institutional and community populations, including the subgroups of chronic mentally ill children and youth, young adult chronic patients, and the homeless chronic mentally ill. Suffice it to note here that although our definition encompasses persons with prolonged moderate-to-severe disability, a significant proportion possess the capacity to live in relative independence if adequate community-based services, social supports, and life opportunities are provided.

REFERENCES

1. Talbott JA (ed): The Chronic Mental Patient: Problems, Solutions, and Recommendations for a Public Policy. Washington, DC, American Psychiatric Association, 1978
2. U.S. Government Accounting Office: Returning the Mentally Disabled to the Community: Government Needs to Do More. Washington, DC, U.S. Government Printing Office, 1977
3. Group for the Advancement of Psychiatry: The Chronic Mental Patient in the Community. New York, Group for the Advancement of Psychiatry, 1978
4. President's Commission on Mental Health: Report of the President's Commission on Mental Health, vol. 1. Washington, DC, U.S. Government Printing Office, 1978
5. Minkoff K: A map of chronic mental patients, in The Chronic Mental Patient: Problems, Solutions, and Recommendations for a Public Policy. Edited by Talbott JA. Washington, DC, American Psychiatric Association, 1978
6. Toward a National Plan for the Chronically Mentally Ill. Report to the Secretary by the Department of Health and Human Services Steering Committee on the Chronically Mentally Ill (DHHS Publication No. (ADM) 81-1077). Rockville, MD, Department of Health and Human Services, 1981
7. Goldman HH, Gattozzi AA, Taube CA: Defining and counting the chronically mentally ill. Hosp Community Psychiatry 32:21–27, 1981
8. Sheehan S: The patient, I: Creedmoor Psychiatric Center. The New Yorker, 25 May 1981, p 49

9. Drake DC: The forsaken. The Philadelphia Inquirer, July 18–24 1982
10. Herman R: One of city's homeless goes home—in death. The New York Times, 31 January 1982
11. Olson WA: Chronic mental illness, what it is and what it means. Wis Med J 80:28–29, 1981
12. Denver Research Institute: Factors Influencing the Deinstitution-alization of the Mentally Ill: A Review and Analysis. Denver, CO, University of Denver, 1981
13. Bachrach LL: Deinstitutionalization: An Analytic Review and Socio-logical Perspective. Rockville, MD, National Institute of Mental Health, 1976
14. Faden VB, Goldman HH: Appropriateness of Placement of Patients in State and County Mental Hospitals. Statistical note 152. Rockville, MD, National Institute of Mental Health, 1979
15. Ashbaugh JW, Leaf PJ, Manderscheid RW, et al: Estimates of the size and selected characteristics of the adult chronically mentally ill population living in U.S. households, in Research in Community and Mental Health, vol. 3. Edited by Greenley J. Greenwich, CN, JAI Press, 1983
16. Von Korff M, Parker RD: The dynamics of the prevalence of chronic episodic disease. Chronic Disease 33:79–85, 1980
17. American Psychiatric Association: Diagnostic and Statistical Manual of Mental Disorders (Third Edition). Washington, DC, American Psychiatric Association, 1980
18. U.S. Department of Health, Education and Welfare: International Classification of Diseases. 8th ed. Washington, DC, U.S. Government Printing Office, 1966
19. Public Law 95-602. Rehabilitation, Comprehensive Services, and Developmental Disabilities Amendments of 1978
20. Grusky O, Tierney K, Manderscheid RW et al: Social bonding and community adjustment of chronically mentally ill adults. J Health Soc Behav 26:49–63, 1985
21. McCarrick AK, Manderscheid RW, Bertolucci DE: Correlates of acting out behavior among the chronically mentally ill. Unpublished paper, 1984
22. Goldman HH, Adams N, Taube CA: Deinstitutionalization data demythologized. Hosp Community Psychiatry 34:129–134, 1983
23. Goldman HH, Taube CA, Regier DA, et al: Multiple functions of the state mental hospital. Am J Psychiatry 140:296–300, 1983
24. Community Support Program: Guidelines. Rockville, MD, National Institute of Mental Health, 1977 (mimeographed)
25. Naierman N: The Chronically Mentally Ill in Community Mental

Health Centers. Washington, DC, Abt Associates, 29 January 1982 (mimeographed)

26. Ashbaugh JW, Hoff MK, Bradley V: Community Support Program Needs Assessment Project: A Review of the Findings in the State CSP Reports and Literature. Boston, Human Services Research Institute, 1980

27. Szymanski HV, Schulberg HC, Salter V et al: Estimating the local prevalence of persons needing community support programs. Hosp Comm Psychiatry 33:370–373, 1982

28. Warheit GJ, Buhl JM, Schwab JJ: Need Assessment Approaches: Concepts and Methods. Department of Health, Education and Welfare publication no. (ADM) 79-472. Rockville, MD, National Institute of Mental Health, 1977

29. Ashbaugh JW: Assessing the need for community supports, in The Chronically Mentally Ill: Assessing Community Support Programs. Edited by Tessler RC, Goldman HH. Cambridge, MA, Ballinger (Harper and Row), 1982, pp 141–158

30. Robins LN: Psychiatric epidemiology. Arch Gen Psychiatry 35:697–702, 1978

31. Weissman MM, Klerman GL: Epidemiology of mental disorders. Arch Gen Psychiatry 35:705–712, 1978

32. Dohrenwend BP, Dohrenwend BS, Gould MS, et al: Scope of the problem. Working paper prepared for the President's Commission on Mental Health, 1978

33. Taylor MA, Abrams R: The prevalence of schizophrenia: a reassessment using modern diagnostic criteria. Am J Psychiatry 135:945–948, 1978

34. Pope HG, Lipinski JF: Diagnosis in schizophrenia and manic-depressive illness. Arch Gen Psychiatry 35:811–827, 1978

35. Carpenter WT, Bartko JJ, Strauss JS, et al: Signs and symptoms as predictors of outcome: a report from the international pilot study of schizophrenia. Am J Psychiatry 135:940–944, 1978

36. Strauss J: Assessment in outpatient settings: the prediction outcome, in The Chronically Mentally Ill: Research and Services. Edited by Mirabi M. New York, SP Medical and Scientific Books, 1984

37. Clayton PJ: The epidemiology of bipolar affective disorder. Compr Psychiatry 22:31–43, 1981

38. Boyd JH, Weissman MM: Epidemiology of affective disorders. Arch Gen Psychiatry 38:1039–1046, 1981

39. Hirschfeld RMA, Cross CK: Epidemiology of affective disorders. Arch Gen Psychiatry 39:35–46, 1982

40. Prien R: Affective disorders, in The Chronically Mentally Ill: Re-

search and Services. Edited by Mirabi M. New York, SP Medical and Scientific Books, 1984

41. Mortimer JA, Schuman L: The Epidemiology of Dementia. New York, Oxford University Press, 1981
42. Brody JA: An epidemiologist views senile dementia—facts and fragments. Am J Epidemiol 115:155–162, 1982
43. Kramer M: The increasing prevalence of mental disorder. Paper presented at Langley Porter Psychiatric Institute, 6 August 1981
44. U.S. Bureau of the Census Survey of Income and Education: Digest of Data on Persons with Disabilities. Washington, DC, Department of Health, Education and Welfare, 1979
45. National Center for Health Statistics: Finding of the 1970 APTD Study. Washington, DC, Social and Rehabilitation Service, 1972
46. Urban Institute: Report of the Comprehensive Service Needs Study. Washington, DC, Department of Health, Education and Welfare, 1975
47. Anderson, JR: Social Security and SSI benefits for the mentally disabled. Hosp Comm Psychiatry 33:295, 1982
48. Goldman HH: Long Term Care for Chronically Mentally Ill. Washington, DC, Urban Institute, 1983
49. Schmidt W, Reinhardt AM, Kane RL, et al: The mentally ill in nursing homes: new back wards in the community. Arch Gen Psychiatry 34:687, 1977
50. Gruenberg E, Archer J: Abandonment of responsibility for the seriously mentally ill. Milbank Memorial Fund 57:485–506, 1979
51. Winslow WW: Changing trends in community mental health centers: keys to survival in the eighties. Hosp Community Psychiatry 33:273–277, 1982
52. Goldman HH, Regier DA, Taube CA, et al: Community mental health centers and the treatment of severe mental disorder. Am J Psychiatry 137:83–86, 1980
53. Langsley DG: The community mental health center: does it treat patients? Hosp Community Psychiatry 31:815–819, 1980
54. Mellody J: Service Delivery Assessment of Boarding Homes. Technical report, region III. Philadelphia, Department of Health and Human Services, 1979
55. Goldman HH: Mental illness and family burden: a public health perspective. Hosp Community Psychiatry 33: 557, 1982
56. Goldman HH: The post-hospital mental patient and family therapy: prospects and populations. Journal of Marital and Family Therapy 6:447, 1980
57. Bachrach LL: Young adult chronic patients: an analytical review of the literature. Hosp Community Psychiatry 33:189, 1982

58. Pepper B, Kirschner MC, Ryglewicz H: The young adult chronic patient: overview of a population. Hosp Community Psychiatry 32:463, 1981

59. Schwartz SR, Goldfinger SM: The new chronic patient: clinical characteristics of an emerging subgroup. Hosp Community Psychiatry 32:470, 1981

60. Taube CA, Thompson JW, Rosenstein MJ, et al: The chronic mental hospital patient. Hosp Community Psychiatry 34:611, 1983

61. Stroup AL, Manderscheid RW: The development of the state mental hospital system in the United States, 1840–1980. Unpublished paper, 1984

62. Woy JR, Goldstrom ID, Manderscheid RW: The young chronic mental patient: report of a national survey. Unpublished paper, 1983

63. Tessler RC, Bernstein AG, Rosen BM et al: The chronically mentally ill in community support systems. Hosp Community Psychiatry 33:208–211, 1982

64. Tessler RC, Goldman HH (eds): The Chronically Mentally Ill: Assessing Community Support Programs. Cambridge, MA, Ballinger (Harper and Row), 1982

65. Tessler RC, Manderscheid RW: Factors affecting adjustment to community living. Hosp Community Psychiatry 33:203, 1982

66. Ashbaugh JW, Leaf PJ, Manderschied RW, et al: Estimates of the size and selected characteristics of the adult chronically mentally ill population living in U.S. households, in Research in Community and Mental Health (Volume 3). Edited by Greenley J. Greenwich, CT, JAI Press, 1982, pp. 3–24

CHAPTER 4

The Homeless Mentally Ill

LEONA L. BACHRACH, PH.D.

OVERVIEW AND SCOPE

Blumer (1) and Stern (2) argue persuasively that objective circumstances do not by themselves constitute a social problem; a subjective definition of the situation as undesirable and socially disruptive is also essential. So it is with the homeless mentally ill. That this population, which is not entirely new, has increased perceptibly in size and visibility in recent years (3) is not sufficient to explain the increased concern of psychiatrists and other mental health professionals. There has also been a growing sense that the individuals in this population somehow epitomize the problems that plague the delivery of services to the chronic mentally ill in the 1980s.

Precisely why this sense of professional responsibility toward the homeless mentally ill has grown in the past six years is not entirely clear, but it is probable that the relative youthfulness of the population and their widespread underuse or inappropriate use of mental health services have been contributing factors. In an undeniable manner, the condition of the homeless mentally ill points to deficits in service delivery for a generation of patients who were to have been the beneficiaries of deinstitutionalized care (4).

In any case, a rapidly growing body of literature, generated by the popular media as well as professional and governmental sources, acknowledges the dimensions of the problems of individuals who are simultaneously homeless and chronically mentally ill. Contributions to that literature differ markedly in their scope, accuracy, and intent. Some pieces represent thoughtful attempts to conceptualize the problems of the homeless mentally ill. Others are reports of painstakingly conceived research efforts. Still others are political in nature and reflect the concerns of various governmental, religious, and social interest groups. It is no exaggeration to say that some are frank diatribes that urge the dispersal, removal, or relocation of the homeless mentally ill.

Yet within this medley there are concordant themes. First, there is a pervasive sense that the homeless mentally ill population is diffcult to pinpoint. A host of conceptual difficulties and confounding variables interfere with efforts to define and count that population with precision.

Second, there are several substantive points of agreement in the literature. It is generally acknowledged that the number of homeless people in the United States is growing steadily (5–7), that their average age is dropping precipitously (8–12), and that the percentage of them who are chronically mentally ill, by any definition, is increasing rapidly (5, 7, 12, 13–16). These circumstances apparently result from the confluence of certain demographic trends and mental health service policies. The coming of age of post-World War II baby boom babies has increased the pool of individuals at risk for chronic mental illnesses. At the same time, public policy relating to the chronic mentally ill, as reflected in deinstitutionalization initiatives and practices, has favored keeping these individuals out of institutional settings and has increased their visibility (3).

Indeed, a third theme running through the literature is that popular, professional, and political sources alike are struggling to establish the relationship between homelessness and mental health service delivery policies. Particular questions concerning the precise contributions of deinstitutionalization to the homeless mentally population recur, as researchers and authors attempt to identify dependent, independent, and intervening variables.

In this chapter I examine these major themes in the literature against the backdrop of my own observations. I have visited numerous facilities for the homeless mentally ill in the United States, Canada, and England, and have discussed problems of service delivery with providers in a variety of settings. In connection with the fact-finding efforts of the American Psychiatric Association's Task Force on the Homeless Mentally Ill (17), I have observed established programs for this population and have also visited other places, where the homeless mentally ill who do not utilize established services congregate. I have attempted, with varying degrees of success, to engage a number of homeless mentally ill people in conversation to try to learn how they perceive their circumstances. These experiences provide an invaluable context within which to interpret the corpus of literature reviewed for this paper.

It must be stressed at the outset that this chapter is not concerned with homeless people in general but seeks instead to focus on those in that population who exhibit the severe psychopathologies that are associated with chronic mental illnesses. This distinction is not uniformly made in all of the literature on the homeless mentally ill. Indeed, some mental health professionals view all homeless people as being at such high risk for mental illness that it is a spurious exercise to differentiate those in the population who have diagnosable illnesses from those who do not.

There is, however, reason to believe that too broad a preoccupation with the entire population of "street people," "bag ladies," "grate gentlemen," and those who are undomiciled for economic or other reasons will ultimately blur the boundaries of social and professional responsibility. Consider this statement by Colman McCarthy (18), a journalist writing in the *Washington Post*:

> The American Psychiatric Association [has] formed a task force . . . to study the homeless and their needs. The studying shouldn't be hard. Church groups, for whom service to the outcast poor is the essence of religion, have opened shelters in all the large cities, and more and more of the small ones. The shelter providers have all the facts and insights the American Psychiatric Association will ever need, beginning with the observation that it shouldn't have taken this long for the doctors to get involved. (p A17)

This quotation, typical of many in the popular media, suggests that psychiatry and the other mental health professions have already been assigned responsibility for the care of homeless people, mentally ill or not. It also implies that unless mental health professionals adopt a proactive stance in stating the limits of their concern, others may assume that task and may, in the process, only confuse and confound the many issues that surround the care of this population.

PROBLEMS IN DELIMITING THE POPULATION

A major problem in defining and counting the population of the homeless mentally ill is that the boundaries of this population are not fixed. It comprises an overlap of two source populations, homeless individuals and the chronically mentally ill, and within each source population, there are shifting subpopulations. The chronic mentally ill, for example, may be found among the residents of state mental hospitals and other psychiatric inpatient facilities, in a variety of community-based residences, in prisons, in temporary shelters, or on the streets. Similarly, the homeless may be found in psychiatric inpatient facilities, in prisons, in temporary shelters, or on the streets. Unknown percentages of both populations move, with varying degrees of regularity, among the different residential settings (19).

Indeed, a host of conceptual and methodologic problems impede efforts to delimit the population of homeless mentally ill individuals. These include difficulties in defining homelessness per se, problems in establishing the presence of psychopathology in a homeless population, overlap of the homeless mentally ill with other populations, heterogeneity within the population, and geographic variability.

Defining Homelessness

That there is no common definition of the homeless mentally ill population will come as no surprise to those who are familiar with the semantics of mental health service planning (20). It is, unfortunately, common practice for words with imprecise definitions and uncertain referents to be used as planning concepts in the mental health field. The concept of the homeless mentally ill is no exception. That population is generally thought to consist of individuals who are simulaneously chronically mentally ill and homeless. However, each of these terms is itself the subject of controversy.

A major deterrent to defining the homeless mentally ill lies in our uncertainty about the precise meaning of homelessness per se. It is widely agreed that homelessness implies both a lack of shelter and a dimension of disaffiliation or social isolation. How, then, should we view migrant farm workers? Does their living in "squalid little camps sometimes five or six in a single room, in barracks or huts that lack basic sanitary facilities" (21) render them homeless? Few professionals would regard living in such circumstances at the pleasure of one's employer as consisting of adequate shelter. In the same vein, it is difficult to say whether members of the Kickapoo Indian tribe who live in reed huts under a bridge across the Rio Grande at Eagle Pass, Texas, are homeless (22). Although these individuals might be viewed as having no permanent shelter, they do have a tribal affiliation. Besides, whether or not a reed hut constitutes shelter in the climate of the Rio Grande Valley is open to question.

Several investigators have actually sought to define homelessness, but their definitions tend to be more descriptive than operational. The Alcohol, Drug Abuse and Mental Health Administration (23) defines the homeless individual as one who lacks shelter, resources, and also community ties. Larew (24) defines homelessness as "a human condition of disaffiliation and detachment . . . from the primary agents of social structure" (p 107).

Even if it were possible to reach consensus on the precise properties of homelessness, however, it would still be difficult to count homeless people. An article in the *San Francisco Bay Guardian* (25) criticizes a police department count of 245 homeless individuals in that city on the grounds that it overlooks the "homeless who hide from them—at least 2,000 more than are publicly sheltered each evening."

The Alcohol, Drug Abuse and Mental Health Administration (23) estimates the total number of homeless persons in the United States to be about two million, with the possibility that as many as half suffer from alcohol, drug abuse, or mental health problems. A more recent and significantly smaller estimate of 250,000 to 350,000 homeless individuals comes from the United States Department of Housing and Urban Development (26). However, the accuracy of the latter estimate has been seriously and responsibly questioned (27–34).

Establishing Psychopathology

In testimony before the New York Governor's Task Force on the Homeless, Kennedy (35) stated: "I recognize and want to emphasize that those individuals who are chronically mentally ill constitute only a percent of those who are homeless, and those who are homeless constitute only a percent of those who are chronically mentally ill." These words imply a second major difficulty in defining and counting the homeless mentally ill. In addition to problems that are associated with defining homelessness per se, there are obvious difficulties in confirming the presence of psychopathology among individuals who are homeless.

In the first place, there are problems associated with the definition of chronicity itself. There has recently been some productive effort to standardize the definition of chronic mental illness, so that the chronic mentally ill are today widely defined as persons with major mental disorders whose illnesses are severe, persistent, and the cause of dysfunction in social and vocational activities (36, 37).

In keeping with geographic shifts in the locus of care in an era of deinstitutionalization, such a definition relies on a combination of diagnostic and functional indicators rather than institutional tenure to establish chronicity. What is still lacking in this definition, however, is consensus on the precise indicators of the severity and persistence of illness and dysfunction.

But even if consensus could be reached about these indicators of chronic mental illness, there would still be special problems associated with identifying chronic mental illness in a homeless population. There are obvious difficulties associated with confirming the presence of psychopathology among individuals who are often reported to be shy and frightened, who frequently abuse alcohol and drugs, and who are likely to have a subculture with different values and norms from those of mental health workers and researchers (38–40).

Baxter and Hopper (41) aptly express concern with the validity of diagnoses made on individuals whose basic subsistence needs are unmet and caution that "were the same individuals to receive several nights of sleep, an adequate diet, and warm social contact, some of their symptoms might subside" (p 402).

It is worth noting parenthetically that homeless people do not necessarily share the definitional problems that mental health professionals seem to have. Those among the homeless who are not mentally ill often appear to be aware of the illnesses of those who are and tend to shun them (41–43). Segal and Baumohl (44), who have studied mentally ill street people in Berkeley, California, refer to them as "space cases," who are "judged by other street people to be delusionary, unpredictable, and unreliable—in the lexicon of the street, 'burned out,' 'fried,' or 'spaced' " (p 358).

Overlap With Other Populations

Problems in defining and counting the homeless mentally ill are further complicated by the overlap of this population with other populations. The characteristics of the homeless mentally ill as a group are not readily distinguishable from those of other chronically mentally ill groups, such as "revolving door" patients (45), "difficult" patients (46–48), "treatment resistant" patients (49), "chronic crisis" patients (50), "urban nomads" (51), and most recently "young adult chronic" patients (52, 53).

In fact, Goldfinger and his colleagues (49) have identified a subgroup of chronic mental patients who fit all of these labels. They are frequent users of emergency and inpatient psychiatric services at San Francisco General Hospital and also of outpatient, residential, and day treatment services. Many of these "acute care recidivists" are also intermittently homeless. In another study of the same population Chafetz and Goldfinger (19) establish that 46 percent of a sample of admissions to psychiatric emergency services were or had at some time been without stable housing, and they conclude that domiciled and undomiciled patients come from a common demographic pool.

This is notable. It suggests strongly that the boundary between the domiciled and undomiciled chronic mentally ill is a very permeable one and that these are probably not two separate populations. Instead, they probably constitute one large population with some rather loose and shifting components.

The homeless mentally ill are also sometimes hard to distinguish from certain populations in jails and correctional facilities (13, 54–57). In an article in the *Washington Post*, Earley (58) asserts that jails have become the "social agencies of last resort" for many chronic mentally ill individuals and that "cuts in social reform programs, hard economic times and the development of psychotropic medicines which have allowed large numbers of disturbed persons to leave mental institutions have contributed to a dramatic increase in persons jailed for non-serious crimes" (p A12). This finding is reinforced by reports in the professional literature. Lamb and Grant (59, 60), for example, write that 36 percent of male and 42 percent of female inmates at Los Angeles County jail facilities, who were referred for psychiatric evaluation, had been living as transients on the streets, on the beach, or in shelters at the time of their arrests.

The homeless mentally ill even overlap to some extent with the population of migrant farm workers. There is documentation in the literature that homeless mentally ill people, at least in some big cities in the East, are at times "shanghaied" into migrant labor streams (41, 61, 62).

Heterogeneity

The homeless mentally ill are frequently difficult to define and count because of the extreme diversity that exists within that population. Like the chronic mentally ill in general (36), homeless mentally ill people do not constitute a uniform population diagnostically, demographically, functionally, or in terms of their residential histories (38, 63–70).

Arce and his colleagues (63, 64) divide the homeless mentally ill population into two groups. "Street people" usually have diagnoses of schizophrenia, substance abuse, or both; a history of hospitalization in a mental hospital; and a variety of health problems. They tend to be floridly psychotic. The "episodic homeless" are usually younger than the street people and tend to have diagnoses of personality disorder, affective disorder, or substance abuse. They tend also to use a wide variety of mental health services sporadically and are likely to be regarded as "difficult" patients. (A third category of homeless individuals described by Arce [63], the "situationally homeless," is identified more by situational stress than by psychopathology. For this population the lack of shelter is generally temporary, and the disaffiliation is less pronounced.)

Nor do the homeless mentally ill constitute a uniform group in terms of appearance. Project HELP (69) in New York City is targeted toward a severely disabled subgroup distinguished by "certain key visual and behavioral characteristics":

> The primary visual indicators include: extremely dirty and dishevelled appearance; obvious lice infestation; torn, dirty and/or layered clothing; weather-inappropriate clothing (especially heavy coats and woolen hats in mid-summer); and a cache of belongings in bags, boxes, shopping carts, etc. The primary behavioral indicators include: walking in traffic, urinating and/or defecating in public, remaining mute and withdrawn. (p 4)

At the opposite pole are individuals described in Reich and Siegel's (12) analysis of recent arrivals to the Bowery in New York City:

> Most of these men are intelligent and have better than the usual education found on the Bowery. They present a fairly intact appearance even when undergoing severe inner disturbance and thus can avoid unwanted hospitalization even when their situation destabilizes and there is a threat of erupting violence. (pp 195–196)

John Hinckley's parents (71) have written that people often find it extremely difficult to accept the presence of severe mental illness in an individual who "looks and acts so 'sane' " (p 3).

Geographic Variability

Finally, it is difficult to define and count the homeless mentally ill because they are often hard to pin down geographically. Although they are frequently associated with inner city residence, members of that population are, as previously noted, found in small cities and suburban and rural areas as well (72–76). Even within cities there are distinctive concentrations of the homeless mentally ill. Barrow and Lovell (38) distinguish between upper west side "street" people and Central Park "park" people in New York City. The latter are characterized by a substantially heavier concentration of males, a markedly higher prevalence of severe psychopathology, and a lower prevalence of substance abuse.

Not only do the homeless mentally ill differ according to where they are; they also vary in how long they have been there. Some are part of an essentially stationary population that is relatively fixed within defined geographic limits, sometimes as small as a few city blocks (24). Others are characterized by extremes of mobility that may cover vast areas.

About 15 years ago Travelers Aid Society (TAS) units throughout the country began to note an upsurge of clients in "psychological flight"

(77). Since then, a number of TAS studies have addressed problems in identifying and serving travelers with severe psychiatric disabilities (78–83). One particularly notable contribution describes a group of severely mentally ill clients identified both in New Orleans and at TAS facilities in other parts of the country. In this population 55 percent were identified in at least one other city, 45 percent in at least three other cities, and 22 percent in at least six other cities in addition to New Orleans (83).

Indeed, migrating homeless mentally ill individuals have been documented in a number of areas, including Arizona (84), California (85, 86), Virginia (87), and Hawaii (88–89). The common finding in all of these reports is summed up in a single sentence in Streltzer's (89) article: "Those who were attempting to escape psychosis continued to be psychotic in Hawaii" (p 468).

NEEDED SERVICES

The service needs of the homeless mentally ill may be broadly broken down into two general categories: those that they share with the domiciled chronic mentally ill and those that are associated with their special undomiciled status.

Service systems for domiciled and undomiciled chronic mentally ill individuals alike must consist of networks of interrelated programs that meet the varied needs of a very heterogeneous and multiply disadvantaged population. Individuals within that population differ widely with respect to demographic indicators, diagnoses, treatment histories, functional levels, residential histories, and prognoses. Although these individuals generally require a wide array of medical, psychiatric, social, rehabilitative, vocational, and case management services, specific service needs vary extensively among local subpopulations. Each local cluster of homeless mentally ill people has its own distinctive demography, epidemiology, and history, as well as its own treatment needs.

In practical terms this means that the mental health service system must not settle for just one modality or approach, because there are too many different kinds of patients who need care. Each community that plans services for the chronic mentally ill, including those who are homeless, must recognize the unique needs of its own target population and must assess the appropriateness of its own resources in meeting those needs. If we have learned one major lesson from three decades of deinstitutionalization, it is that there is no single right way, or place, in which to serve these patients.

Service systems for the homeless mentally ill, like those for other chronic mentally ill individuals, should contain screening and referral services, crisis stabilization services, a comprehensive array of treatment settings, a network of treatment services, transportation services, and information and evaluation services (90). Since these components are described at some length in the literature on the chronic mentally ill, I shall not elaborate upon them here.

However, it is critical to note that each of these service categories should be considered as a separate entity in the planning process. A tendency to think of them interchangeably has often been detrimental to the welfare of chronic mentally ill individuals. This is particularly true with respect to the frequent confusion of residential and treatment settings, as illustrated by the concept of the least-restrictive environment: residence outside of an institution does not by itself guarantee a lessening of restrictiveness in other aspects of patients' lives (91). Thus, recognition that these two functions are distinct must guide the planning process.

Indeed, the confusion of residential and treatment settings has had particularly powerful consequences for the homeless mentally ill (92). It is not unusual for planners to think of the residential needs of these individuals but to ignore their various treatment needs, including their frequent requirements for medical and psychiatric care (41, 64, 93–95).

There are additional considerations to note in planning services that are specific to the needs of the undomiciled members of the chronic mentally ill population. Comprehensive care, a concept much in vogue in service planning, has unique connotations for these individuals, who generally have nothing and need everything. In keeping with the complex nature of homelessness—it is more than a simple lack of shelter—Barrow and Lovell (38) list some 70 separate services that homeless mentally ill people often need, including some not very traditional ones, such as providing a mailbox where Supplemental Security Income (SSI) checks can be delivered, delousing, and showering. Gilliam (96) has a sobering piece in the *Washington Post* about an increase in surgical amputations for frostbite among the homeless mentally ill.

Providers may be hard pressed to ensure required services in their facilities, since organized mental health programs are generally not prepared to respond to patients' basic subsistence and sanitary needs. Until these have been fulfilled, however, clinical and rehabilitative efforts will probably have little positive effect.

Finally, in assessing the service needs of the homeless mentally ill, careful attention must once again be paid to conceptual considerations (97). Some researchers and service providers are concerned with the prevalence of mental illness in homeless populations. They want to know, in effect, how may homeless people are chronically mentally ill. But others seek guidance from a completely different vantage point. They turn the question around and examine the prevalence of homelessness among the chronic mentally ill: they want to know, in effect, how many chronic mentally ill people have no place to live. These are two basically different approaches to studying the homeless mentally ill population, and each entails different case-finding procedures and needs assessment methodologies.

Adopting one or another of these approaches in service planning is likely to have far-reaching implications for policy formulation. Planning that proceeds from the determination of chronic mental illness among homeless people will probably be concerned with aggressive methods for engaging individuals who have eluded the service system. Contrariwise, planning that proceeds from the determination of homelessness among people who are chronically mentally ill is more likely to focus on the "cracks" through which the chronic mentally ill are said to fall and on such pragmatic concerns as the differential effects of various discharge planning policies on members of that population. It is well for planners and service planners to be aware of these differences lest they find themselves consulting needs assessment studies that have answers for questions other than those they wish to ask.

BARRIERS TO CARE

The homeless mentally ill tend to experience today's mental health service system as a series of paradoxes defying ready solution (98). They generally encounter severe impediments to care. These barriers fall into several interrelated broad categories: preclusive admission policies, inadequate services, geographically determined responsibility, inappropriate expectations, and social distance.

Preclusive Admission Policies

Specific services for the homeless mentally ill, like those for other chronically mentally ill individuals, are often targeted toward the best-functioning members of that population. The result is that programs may be totally unavailable to those who need services most. A newspaper article describes a suburban community outside of Washington, D.C., for example, as having a "fledging supervised-apartment program and a group home for the mentally ill, but only for those who have been judged capable of being rehabilitated, not for the so-called hopeless cases" (99). This kind of planning, which is not uncommon, skews service provision away from the homeless mentally ill population, which is disproportionately characterized by poorly functioning individuals.

That such preclusive admission policies flourish should come as no surprise. Service planners and providers may be expected to do what they know how to do—to treat those who best respond to their interventions; and better-functioning individuals must not be abandoned simply because the "answers" to caring for the most disturbed are so elusive. Exclusionary policies are, moreover, reinforced by certain attitude sets of service providers. Not only does the stigma of working with the most severely ill influence gate-keeping behavior, but service providers tend to measure their effectiveness in terms of "cures" for their patients (100).

Other preclusive admission policies result from a failure on the part of service planners to perceive accurately the program needs of the population they are attempting to serve. There is often a time lag between the identification of service needs and the implementation of programs directed toward the needs. In the case of the chronic mentally ill, that lag is manifested in initiatives designed for earlier generations of institutionalized patients. "Aftercare," assisting long-time residents of institutions to adapt to life in the community, is a fundamental program planning concept today. Yet an aftercare focus denies the essentially noninstitutional cast of today's chronic mentally ill population and overlooks the existence of a rapidly growing portion of that population that has never had hospitalizations of any kind. Many of these individuals are homeless (52, 101).

Inadequate Services

Very often specific services that the homeless mentally ill require simply do not exist as part of the mental health service system's offerings. One reason for this deficit is that, as noted above, the homeless mentally ill tend to have service needs that are extraordinary both in number and in content. In addition, the absence of adequate services may also result from a failure in concept. Planners often view alternatives for the homeless mentally ill simplistically—as if, perhaps, increasing available shelter space will by itself take care of their needs. Having a place to sleep is an obvious and essential requirement for homeless mentally ill individuals, but failure to recognize their other needs denies the complexity of their circumstances.

Related to oversimplification is a tendency to view the needs of the homeless mentally ill in absolute terms (102). In the well-chosen words of Baxter and Hopper (103), service planning for these individuals is frequently a "Hobson's choice which depicts options as either mental hospitalization or a life on the streets" (p 58). Yet many who spend time with this population are adamant in their conviction that there are shades in between these two extremes and that more moderate options are both viable and necessary (103).

The very existence of the homeless mentally ill is often denied, and there is a widespread tendency either to ignore these individuals altogether so that they stay hidden from view, or else, in the name of "humanity," to "dump" them—to shunt them into places that ignore the specificity and the breach of their needs. This is evident in the way that shelter facilities are frequently used for this population. Bassuk (65) aptly points out that even those shelters that admit mentally ill individuals (and not all shelters do) are usually not connected with clinical services and thus stand outside the spectrum of linked psychiatric programs within a given community. Such service isolation contradicts established principles of effective planning for the chronic mentally ill (90).

Geographically Determined Responsibility

Historically, one of the major philosophic underpinnings of the community mental health movement involved the fixing of responsibility for chronic mental patients within defined geographical areas (104). Although such "catchmenting" is no longer discussed extensively in the literature, its original intent, to force providers to assume responsibility for the care of individuals within circumscribed boundaries so that no one would be overlooked (105), continues to influence service provision.

For the homeless mentally ill, geographically determined responsibility has backfired. In order to qualify for care in many service settings, chronic mental patients must meet a variety of residence requirements. Obviously, such a policy imposes severe barriers to care for people who have no home and no fixed address.

Residence-based requirements for eligibility also often affect the ability of many homeless individuals to qualify for social service and medical treatment entitlements (65, 98, 106, 107). Segal and his colleagues (101) note that the lack of a permanent address "greatly increases the likelihood that an individual's SSI application will not be processed" (p 398). Even if the application is processed, the applicant may still experience difficulty in receiving entitlements, because "notification of psychiatric appointments, requests for additional information or release forms, and all other communications from the Social Security Office are routinely conducted by mail" (101).

It may be noted parenthetically that, despite the emphasis on geographic responsibility, there are times when the homeless mentally ill are actively excluded from their communities (103). Wealthy suburbs sometimes refer seriously ill citizens to inner city agencies (108). Whether those referrals are actually completed is questionable. In addition, some communities are known to utilize "Greyhound therapy," the practice of providing homeless mentally ill people with one-way bus tickets out of town (86, 109), thereby reinforcing the heavy mobility of much of this population.

Inappropriate Expectations

The homeless mentally ill are often further impeded in their access to mental health services by unrealistic expectations on the part of planners and service providers. The current controversy over whether individuals are homeless by "choice"(110) reflects a naive expectation that those who are chronically mentally ill share the same expectations and prospects as other members of society. However, illness itself may often intervene to limit the choices of the homeless mentally ill (31, 40, 111–113).

Some investigators conclude that there is a great need for highly structured treatment settings where homeless mentally ill individuals can receive at least a minimum of attention and will not be exposed to the uncertainties and rigors of street life (59, 60). However, the needs of individuals who require this kind of structure stand in direct contrast to societal and professional norms that encourage freedom for the mentally ill and define that freedom on the basis of individuals' consent to be placed in "restrictive" treatment settings. Often, homeless mentally ill people are unwilling or unable to give that consent (13, 65, 106, 114–116).

However, not all the homeless mentally ill are necessarily in need of structured treatment settings. Barrow and Lovell (38) write that there is a need for *less* structure than is generally offered in services for much of this population, and they support the use of drop-in centers operated by a staff specially skilled in working with homeless people. Segal and Baumohl (44) concur in this view.

The two positions regarding structure noted here, though polarized, are not necessarily contradictory, for the homeless mentally ill are a diverse population, and different individuals in it have different service needs. What both of these viewpoints point up is a frequent failure on the part of service planners and providers to plan a realistic array of service structures for the target population and to assess, on an individualized basis, the appropriate placement of those who utilize their services.

Social Distance

Closely related to the inconsistency between professionals' expectations and many homeless mentally ill individuals' capabilities is a paradox created by the fact that, for all practical purposes, they live in different worlds. The homeless mentally ill tend to have a unique cultural identity and a limited universe of discourse with those who attempt to serve them (101, 117, 118). Their respective values differ, and certainly the norms that govern their behavior are often disparate. Baxter and Hopper (119) provide forceful documentation of the existence of a separate culture among homeless street people, a culture that often escapes the notice of those who provide them with services.

Larew (24) explains the social distance paradox:

> An inability . . . on the part of the homeless individual to live in a traditional lifestyle poses a special problem for the traditional service providers and for the community planners that offer services to transients. Traditional services are geared toward either religious evangelism or rehabilitation, with an emphasis on gaining employable skills. These two goals conflict with the transients' inability to look beyond the next meal or bed. Workers who deliver the services often place the highest value on the client who least fulfills the transient criteria. The transient who most frequently needs a variety of services is left unattended. (p 109)

Carried to extremes, this kind of cultural bias may result in public policy that denies basic necessities to the homeless mentally ill on the assumption that their failure to look after themselves bespeaks a disinclination to "earn" their keep and an eagerness to acquire unneeded, and undeserved, handouts (120–122).

THE ROLE OF DEINSTITUTIONALIZATION

Like other chronic mentally ill people, those who are homeless have been profoundly affected by deinstitutionalization—by its policies, its practices, and its priorities (12, 102, 123–129). However, the barriers discussed above suggest that those among the chronic mentally ill who are undomiciled have a special relationship to deinstitutionalization in that the benefits of that basically humanistic movement have largely eluded them. Usually unable to surmount barriers to care, these individuals have fallen prey to homelessness. Once homeless, they usually have not had the resources needed to escape that status (130–132). Although they are often geographically mobile, they lack the personal and social resources— the constellation of attributes that Segal and his colleagues (101) call "social margin"—to be vertically mobile; that is, to become something other than what they are.

Most analyses of the homeless mentally ill readily acknowledge the contribution of deinstitutionalization to their plight. However, in the special "numbers game" atmosphere in which mental health service planning often occurs, there are occasional suggestions that the number of deinstitutionalized people among the homeless is actually quite small and is growing even smaller as state mental hospital populations continue to shrink.

Such thinking takes an extremely simplistic view of both deinstitutionalization and homelessness. If the number of chronic mentally ill individuals released from state mental hospitals is supplemented by the number of persons who have never been institutionalized precisely *because* of so-called "admission diversion" policies in many service systems (133–137), a different picture emerges. Many never-institutionalized individuals are homeless because in today's system of care they have no place to go. They do not even fit into aftercare residential programs because they fail to qualify for aftercare, because they have never been in state hospitals in the first place—a vicious circle that is becoming increasingly difficult to penetrate.

In short, one who is mentally ill and homeless need not necessarily ever have been institutionalized in order to be affected by deinstitutionalization: the policies and initiatives of the deinstitutionalization movement so pervade service planning today that they affect even patients who have never had institutional stays. Whatever their treatment histories, today's homeless mentally ill are, as a group, essentially deinstitutionalized persons, for they must seek treatment and support in service systems that are themselves primarily deinstitutionalized. Thus, it is deinstitutionalization that gives substance to their problems in receiving adequate care.

SERVICE AND PLANNING TRENDS

The problems detailed in this paper may well lead to pessimism, to the sense that there are no possible solutions to meeting the service needs of the homeless mentally ill. Yet, from another perspective, it may be suggested that our very ability to summarize and analyze service delivery issues presupposes the development of a body of relevant knowledge. Thus, even though our service structures for the homeless mentally ill are inadequate, and even though our efforts to reach individuals in that population are frequently misdirected, we now have an understanding of some basic requisites of appropriate planning, and these are increasingly being incorporated into targeted services.

More and more today the proverbial cracks through which chronic mental patients are said to fall are being explored. James (138) has written that needs assessments in community mental health planning must begin with the study of waiting lists and other indicators of service backups. Surely there are few events that point to backups and hiatuses more eloquently than does the growth of a population whose members, in the wake of deinstitutionalization, find themselves without homes, without treatment, and without community supports.

A major service gap, of course—indeed, the most apparent one—is in the area of shelter. Fortunately, there is a growing appreciation today that there is no single kind of residential setting that equally fulfills the needs of all homeless mentally ill persons. This has prompted an increased emphasis on including a variety of residential alternatives among services for the homeless mentally ill. Different members of that population have different kinds of housing requirements, and they need residential settings that range from places where they may live in relative independence to highly structured long-term care settings.

But providing adequate housing is only a starting point (124), and the trend toward individualized placement is emerging in other service areas as well. Indeed, the development of differentiated treatment settings for the homeless mentally ill (139) is consistent with the notion that individualized programming is an essential part of treatment for the chronic mentally ill in general, whether the specific intervention offered is chemotherapy, psychotherapy, psychosocial rehabilitation, or some combination of these or other treatment modalities. For the homeless in that population, individualized programming is particularly critical because of their fearfulness, resistance, and general inaccessibility.

Some homeless mentally ill persons may be persuaded to seek treatment in loosely structured, informal, "no questions asked" *drop-in centers.* The attractiveness of these programs is generally thought to be enhanced when they offer a variety of services. Thus, those centers that offer shelter and food in addition to socialization and rehabilitation opportunities have an increased chance of responding to the needs of at least some members of the homeless mentally ill population. And those that provide on-site medical, dental, or psychiatric care have even greater relevance.

There are, however, many among the homeless mentally ill who will not volunteer to visit a drop-in center, no matter how informal and how nonthreatening the milieu. Some of these individuals may perhaps be reached through *outreach programs* whose workers make aggressive contact with members of the target population by frequenting those places, often hidden, where they live (140). Mobile vans are often part of the basic equipment of outreach programs.

Because of their nature, outreach programs must necessarily offer a narrower range of services than drop-in centers. Frequently, they concentrate on dispensing food, making referrals, and transporting individuals to emergency or other services. The distinguishing aspect of these programs is that they make a point of going to patients instead of expecting the patients to come to them, a necessary circumstance for many of the more withdrawn in the population. Indeed, outreach workers must often be prepared to spend many months of protracted initial, noninvasive contact with particular homeless individuals before they are able to establish enough trust to communicate with them. It may even take multiple encounters before an individual member of the population will accept an offer of food, which frequently serves as basic currency for establishing communication between a worker and a homeless mentally ill person.

Shelters, both transitional and permanent, and *soup kitchens* generally provide services to the homeless mentally ill at specific times of the day or night. Sometimes both shelter and food services are combined in a single setting. Such basic subsistence programs, while of fundamental importance in responding to the survival needs of the homeless mentally ill, are, however, increasingly being viewed as stop-gap measures. There is a developing consensus that they do go far enough in ensuring comprehensive care to a multiply disabled population with definite and marked medical, psychiatric, social, and vocational service needs. Accordingly, there is a trend toward not isolating these substance functions but rather attempting to provide them in multiservice settings.

The emergence of differentiated service structures is being accompanied by an expansion of service-oriented research on the homeless mentally ill (141). Through a variety of needs assessment, epidemiologic, and program evaluation studies, an increased effort is now being made to use documented findings to inform the planning process, and a partnership between planning and research is beginning to evolve. Pioneering work in this effort has been performed at the New York State Psychiatric Institute (38, 39, 106).

Finally, there is evidence that the delivery of services to the homeless mentally ill is emerging, at least in some communities, as a field of cooperative enterprise (142), particularly between church-affiliated organizations and mental health service agencies. The leadership role in caring for homeless persons that has traditionally been assumed by selected religious organizations (18, 143) is increasingly being carried over to the specialized needs of the undomiciled chronic mentally ill. Thus, as members of the mental health professions seek to develop new skills to apply in the care of this population, they are more and more often doing so in climates where more than mere lip service is given to the necessity for interagency communication and cooperation. Indeed, combining specialized mental health expertise with the unique dimensions of charity and acceptance that are the hallmarks of many church-related programs is generating a new kind of service delivery climate, one that appears to hold great benefits for the homeless mentally ill in many communities (142, 144–147).

CONCLUSIONS

It is entirely appropriate for a conference on the chronic mental patient in 1984 to investigate issues concerning the provision of services to those who are simultaneously homeless and chronically mentally ill. Whether they are intermittently or permanently undomiciled, the homeless mentally ill serve to place in bold relief those service delivery problems that are typical of chronic mental patients: they are impeded from access to care by the absence of a comprehensive array of basic services, by the difficulties associated with implementing continuity of their care, and by uncertainty regarding their status as rightful recipients of services.

In addition, the homeless mentally ill experience a series of special service delivery problems that are related to their undomiciled status. They often find themselves trapped in circumstances that afford them little hope.

Our knowledge of how to overcome barriers in the care of the homeless mentally ill is imperfect. It is not surprising that we still have much to learn. The Director of Policy Studies of the Health and Welfare Council of Central Maryland has summarized the situation by noting, in a Public Television interview, that the homeless mentally ill "didn't get sick in a day, and they won't get well in a day" (148).

We do know, however, that effective care for this population must acknowledge the unique interaction of chronicity and homelessness. Adapting principles of effective care to the special concerns of the homeless portion of the chronic mentally ill population is emerging as a major service planning challenge for the second half of the 1980s.

REFERENCES

1. Blumer H: Social problems as collective behavior. Social Problems 18:298–306, 1971
2. Stern MJ: The emergence of the homeless as a public problem. Social Service Review, June 1984, pp 291–301
3. Bachrach LL: The homeless mentally ill and mental health services: an analytical review of the literature, in The Homeless Mentally Ill: A Task Force Report of the American Psychiatric Association. Edited by Lamb HR. Washington, DC, American Psychiatric Association, 1984

4. Bachrach LL: An overview of deinstitutionalization, in Deinstitutionalization. Edited by Bachrach LL. New Directions for Mental Health Services, no. 18. San Francisco, Jossey-Bass, 1983
5. Hayes RN: Reforming current city policies. CBC Quarterly 2:1–4, 1982
6. Herman R: City's homeless: story of Bobby Cruz. The New York Times, 19 November 1979, pp B1, B4
7. U.S. Senate: Special Hearing on Street People. Washington, DC, U.S. Government Printing Office, 1983
8. Leaf A, Cohen M: Providing Services for the Homeless: The New York City Program. New York, City of New York Human Resources Administration, December 1982
9. Multnomah County: The Homeless Poor 1984. Portland, OR, 1984
10. New York State Office of Mental Health: Who Are the Homeless? A Study of Randomly Selected Men Who Use the New York City Shelters. Albany, NY, May 1982
11. Prevost JA: Youthful chronicity: paradox of the 80s. Hosp Community Psychiatry 33:173, 1982
12. Reich R, Siegel L: The emergency of the Bowery as a psychiatric dumping ground. Psychiatr Q 50:191–201, 1978
13. Drake DC: The forsaken. The Philadelphia Inquirer, 18–24 July 1982
14. Governor's Select Commission on the Future of the State-Local Mental Health System: Report of the Subcommittee on the New York City Psychiatric Bed Crisis. Albany, December 1983
15. Left out in the cold. Time, 19 December 1983, pp 14–15
16. U.S. Department of Health and Human Services and U.S. Department of Housing and Urban Development: Report of Federal Efforts to Respond to the Shelter and Basic Living Needs of Chronically Mentally Ill Individuals. Washington, DC, February 1983 (photocopied)
17. Lamb HR (ed): The Homeless Mentally Ill: A Task Force Report of the American Psychiatric Association. Washington, DC, American Psychiatric Association, 1984
18. McCarthy C: A doctor's house call on the homeless. The Washington Post, 5 November 1983, p A17
19. Chafetz L, Goldfinger SM: Residential instability in a psychiatric emergency setting. Psychiatr Q 56:20–34, 1984
20. Bachrach LL: Slogans and euphemisms: the functions of semantics in MHMR care. Special lecture presented to the Texas Department of Mental Health and Mental Retardation. Austin, 22 October, 1984
21. Sinclair W: Needed workers are caught in the stream. The Washington Post, 23 August 1981, pp A1, A18

22. "Lost" Indian tribe seeks recognition and a home. The New York Times, 26 December, 1981, p 12
23. Alcohol, Drug Abuse and Mental Health Administration: Alcohol, Drug Abuse and Mental Health Problems of the Homeless. Rockville MD, Alcohol, Drug Abuse and Mental Health Administration, 1983
24. Larew BI: Strange strangers: serving transients. Social Casework 63:107–113, 1980
25. Ross J: The homeless are still with us. San Francisco Bay Guardian, 7 December 1983, p 9–13
26. U.S. Department of Housing and Urban Development: A Report to the Secretary on the Homeless and Emergency Shelters. Washington, DC, HUD, 1984
27. Goode WW: HUD and the homeless. The Washington Post, 20 May 1984, p B7
28. Guillermoprieto A: Report on the homeless attacked in Hill hearing. The Washington Post, 25 May 1984, p A15
29. Harris M: Counting the homeless in S.F. San Francisco Chronicle, 3 May 1984, p 8
30. Kurtz H: HUD says number of U.S. homeless falls well below private estimates. The Washington Post, 2 May 1984, p A2
31. McCarthy C: Reagan's grate society. The Washington Post, 11 February 1984, p A23
32. McCarthy C: Just what the homeless needed. The Washington Post, 12 May 1984, p A15
33. Pear R: Homeless in U.S. put at 250,000: far less than previous estimates. The New York Times, 2 May 1984, pp A1, A20
34. The U.S. Senate: HUD Report on Homelessness. Washington, DC, U.S. Government Printing Office, 1984
35. Kennedy C: Testimony before Governor's Task Force on the Homeless. New York City, 23 April 1983
36. Goldman HH, Gattozzi AA, Taube CA: Defining and counting the chronically mentally ill. Hosp Community Psychiatry 32:21–27, 1981
37. Peele R, Palmer RR: Patient rights and patient chronicity. Journal of Psychiatry and Law, Spring 1980, pp 59–71
38. Barrow S, Lovell AM: Evaluation of Project Reach Out, 1981–82. New York, New York State Psychiatric Institute, 30 June 1982 (photocopied)
39. Barrow S, Lovell AM: CSS preliminary report. New York, New York State Psychiatric Institute, 15 April 1983 (photocopied)
40. du Buclet L: Seeking out the homeless. The Washington Post, 8 March 1984, p C3
41. Baxter E, Hopper K: The new mendicancy: homeless in New York City. Am J Orthopsychiatry 54:393–408, 1982

42. McGrory M: State of union seems less rosy at a shelter for the homeless. The Washington Post, 26 January 1984, p A2

43. Robinson E: Down on his luck. The Washington Post, 29 April 1984, p B8

44. Segal SP, Baumohl J: Engaging the disengaged: proposals on madness and vagrancy. Social Work 25:358–365, 1980

45. Geller MP: The "revolving door": a trap or a life style? Hosp Community Psychiatry 33:388–389, 1982

46. Neill JR: The difficult patient: identification and response. J Clin Psychiatry 40:209–212, 1979

47. Robbins E, Stern M, Robbins L, et al: Unwelcome patients: where can they find asylum? Hosp Community Psychiatry 29:44–46, 1978

48. White HS: Managing the difficult patient in the community residence, in Issues in Community Residential Care. Edited by Budson R. New Directions for Mental Health Services, no. 11. San Francisco, Jossey-Bass, 1981

49. Goldfinger SM, Hopkin JT, Surber RW: Treatment resisters or system resisters? Toward a better service system for acute care recidivists, in Advances in Treating the Young Adult Chronic Patient. Edited by Pepper B, Ryglewicz H. New Directions for Mental Health Services, no. 21. San Francisco, Jossey-Bass, 1984

50. Bassuk E, Gerson S: Chronic crisis patients: a discrete clinical group. Am J Psychiatry 137:1513–1517, 1980

51. Appleby L, Slagg N, Desai PN: The urban nomad: a psychiatric problem, in Current Psychiatric Therapies, vol. 21. Edited by Masserman JH. New York, Grune and Stratton, 1982

52. Bachrach LL: Young adult chronic patients: an analytical review of the literature. Hosp Community Psychiatry 33:189–197, 1982

53. Pepper B, Kirshner MC, Ryglewicz H: The young adult chronic patient: overview of a population. Hosp Community Psychiatry 32:463–469, 1981

54. Elsner M: Do Tucsonians really think the mentally ill belong in jail? Tucson [Arizona] Citizen, 4 February 1983

55. Elsner M: Jail—a poor housing alternative for the mentally ill. AMISA [Alliance for the Mentally Ill of Southern Arizona] Newsletter, February/March 1984, p 2

56. Stelovich S: From the hospital to the prison: a step forward in deinstitutionalization? Hosp Community Psychiatry 30:618–620, 1979

57. White RD: Mentally ill, retarded suffer in crowded jails. The Washington Post, 19 November 1981, pp Md.1, Md.7

58. Earley P: Jails are becoming "dumping grounds," federal government advisory panel told. The Washington Post, 17 June 1983, p A12

59. Lamb HR, Grant HW: The mentally ill in an urban county jail. Arch Gen Psychiatry 39:17–22, 1982
60. Lamb HR, Grant RW: Mentally ill women in a county jail. Arch Gen Psychiatry 40:362–368, 1983
61. Henry N: The long, hot wait for pickin' work. The Washington Post, 9 October 1983, pp A1, A16
62. Herman R: Some freed mental patients make it, some do not. The New York Times, 19 November 1979, pp B1, B4
63. Arce AA: Statement before the Committee on Appropriations, in U.S. Senate Special Hearing on Street People. Washington, DC, U.S. Government Printing Office, 1983
64. Arce AA, Tadlock M, Vergare MH, et al.: A psychiatric profile of street people admitted to an emergency shelter. Hosp Community Psychiatry 34:812–817, 1983
65. Bassuk EL: Addressing the needs of the homeless. Boston Globe Magazine, 6 November 1983, pp 12, 60ff
66. Kaplan JL: Homeless, hungry and Jewish. Washington Jewish Week, 16 February 1984, pp 1, 4–5
67. Lipton F, Sabatini A, Katz S: Down and out in the city: the homeless mentally ill. Hosp Community Psychiatry 34:818–821, 1983
68. Down and out in America. Newsweek, 15 March 1982, pp 28–29
69. Project HELP Summary, October 30, 1982–August 31, 1983. New York State Community Support Services, Gouverneur Hospital, New York City, 1983 (photocopied)
70. Rousseau AM: Shopping Bag Ladies. New York, Pilgrim Press, 1981
71. Hinckley J, Hinckley J: Illness is the culprit! Reader's Digest: March 1983, pp 27, 31
72. Bachrach LL: Psychiatric services in rural areas: a sociological overview. Hosp Community Psychiatry 34:215–226, 1983
73. Fishman C: Homeless in Fairfax lose shelter. The Washington Post, 1 April 1984, pp B1, B4
74. Melton RH: Shelter gives life to down and out. The Washington Post, 23 December 1983, pp C1, C7
75. Mintz J: Arlington shuts facility for homeless. The Washington Post, 16 February 1984, p C4
76. Young BJ: Testimony, in Homelessness in America: Hearing before the Subcommittee on Housing and Community Development, U.S. House of Representatives, December 15, 1982. Washington, DC, U.S. Government Printing Office, 1983, pp 148–151
77. New tasks faced by Travelers Aid. The New York Times, 4 May 1969, p 53
78. Goldberg M: The runaway Americans. Mental Hygiene 56:13–21, 1972

79. Green C: The Transient Mentally Disabled: A New Challenge to Travelers Aid Services. San Francisco, Travelers Aid Society, 1978

80. Health and Welfare Council of Central Maryland: A Report to the Greater Baltimore Shelter Network on Homelessness in Central Maryland. Baltimore, June 1983

81. Lewis N: Community Intake Services for the Transient Mentally Disabled (TMD). Travelers Aid Society of San Francisco, 1978 (photocopied)

82. Smith HA: Psycho-social development of flight chronic patients. New Orleans, Travelers Aid Society, 1980 (photocopied)

83. Travelers Aid Society of Greater New Orleans: Summary of Study of Wandering Mentally Ill, Travelers Aid Society, 1976 (photocopied)

84. Brown C, MacFarlane S, Paredes R, et al: The Homeless of Phoenix: Who Are They? And What Should Be Done? Phoenix South Community Mental Health Center, 1983

85. Farr RK: Skid Row Project. Los Angeles County Department of Mental Health, 18 January 1982 (photocopied)

86. van Winkle WA: Bedlam by the bay. New West, 1 December 1980, pp 81–89

87. Chmiel AJ, Akhtar S, Morris J: The long-distance psychiatric patient in the emergency room. Int J Soc Psychiatry 25:38–46, 1979

88. Kimura SP, Mikolashek PL, Kirk SA: Madness in paradise: psychiatric crises among newcomers in Honolulu. Hawaii Medical J 34:275–278, 1975

89. Strelzer J: Psychiatric emergencies in travelers to Hawaii. Compr Psychiatry 20:463–468, 1979

90. Bachrach LL: Planning services for chronically mentally ill patients. Bull Menninger Clin 47:163–188, 1983

91. Bachrach LL: Is the least restrictive environment always the best? Sociological and semantic implications. Hosp Community Psychiatry 31:97–103, 1980

92. McGerigle P, Lauriat A: More Than Shelter: A Community Response to Homelessness. Boston, United Community Planning Corporation and Massachusetts Association for Mental Health, 1983

93. Goodwin M: Koch considers using ships as shelter for homeless. The New York Times, 28 April 1984, p 27

94. Greening of Skid Row. Time, 19 July 1982, p 81

95. Rule S: Outlook for homeless ill called grim. The New York Times, 29 October 1983, p 31

96. Gilliam D: Amputees. The Washington Post, 12 March 1984, p B1

97. Bachrach LL: Interpreting research on the homeless mentally ill: some caveats. Hosp Community Psychiatry 35:914–917, 1984

98. Homeless in America. Newsweek, 2 January 1984, pp 20–29
99. Sugawara S: Mentally ill often are left on their own in Fairfax. The Washington Post, 20 November 1983, pp B1, B2
100. Stern R, Minkoff K: Paradoxes in programming for chronic patients in a community clinic. Hosp Community Psychiatry 30:613–617, 1979
101. Segal SP, Baumohl J, Johnson E: Falling through the cracks. Mental disorder and social margin in a young vagrant population. Social Problems 24:387–400, 1977
102. Goleman D: Lawsuits try to force care for the mentally ill. The New York Times, 24 April 1984, pp C1, C10
103. Baxter E, Hopper K: Troubled on the streets: the mentally disabled, homeless poor, in The Chronic Mental Patient: Five Years Later. Edited by Talbott JA. Orlando, FL, Grune and Stratton, 1984
104. Group for the Advancement of Psychiatry: Community Psychiatry: A Reappraisal. New York, Group for the Advancement of Psychiatry, 1983
105. Panzetta A: Community Mental Health: Myth and Reality. Philadelphia, Lea and Febiger, 1971
106. Barrow S, Lovell AM: Evaluation of the Referral of Outreach Clients to Mental Health Services, Private Homes for Adults, CSS Eligibility, and the Acute Day Hospitals. New York, New York State Psychiatric Institute, 30 June 1983
107. Christmas and food lines. The Washington Post, 25 December 1983, p B6
108. Muscatine A: Suburbs send homeless to D.C. shelters. The Washington Post, 19 February 1983, pp A1, A31
109. Cordes C: The plight of the homeless mentally ill. APA Monitor, February 1984, pp 1, 13
110. Williams J: Homeless choose to be, Reagan says. The Washington Post, 1 February 1984, pp A1, A4
111. Homeless by choice? The New York Times, 7 February 1984, p A24
112. Raspberry W: Homeless by choice. The Washington Post, 3 February 1984, p A19
113. Schanberg SH: Reagan's homeless. The New York Times, 4 February 1984, p 23
114. Kamen A: The right to refuse treatment. The Washington Post, 20 May 1982, pp B1, B4
115. Quindlen A: About New York. The New York Times, 15 December 1982, p B3
116. Sullivan R: New York to give funds to operate 15 mental clinics. The New York Times, 23 November 1983

117. O'Connor J: Sheltering the homeless in the nation's capital. Hosp Community Psychiatry 34:863, 879

118. Sullivan R: Officials say that homeless often refuse aid from city. The New York Times, 22 October 1983

119. Baxter E, Hopper K. Private Lives/Public Spaces: Homeless Adults on the Streets of New York City. New York, Community Service Society, 1981

120. Engel M, Sargent ED: Meese's hunger remarks stir more outrage among groups. The Washington Post, 11 December 1983, pp A1, A10

121. Meese E: The food is free and . . . that's easier than paying for it. The Washington Post, 10 December 1983, p A2

122. Raspberry W: Garbage eaters. The Washington Post, 2 May 1984, p A21

123. Dupwe RL: Refugees on the grates. The Washington Post, 2 January 1983, p B6

124. Evans S: Experts tell D.C. panel the homeless need aid. The Washington Post, 21 November 1984, p A7

125. Gershberg JM: Homeless in New York. The Pharos, Fall 1983, pp 7–10

126. Goldsmith MF: From mental hospitals to jails: the pendulum swings. JAMA 250:3017–3019

127. Jones RE: Street people and psychiatry: an introduction. Hosp Community Psychiatry 34:807–811, 1983

128. Krucoff C: Psychiatrist of the streets. The Washington Post, 24 May 1984, pp D1, D15

129. Lyons RD: How release of mental patients began. The New York Times, 30 October 1984, pp C1, C4

130. Carmody D: City to spend $100 million on homeless. The New York Times, 10 October 1984, pp A1, B4

131. De Wolfe E: Skid row: hotels vanishing as living space for 10,000 people. Los Angeles Times, 26 April 1982

132. Schanberg SH: Emptying and gentrifying. The New York Times, 23 October 1984, p A33

133. Dionne EJ: Mental patient cutbacks planned. The New York Times, 8 December 1978, p B3

134. Morrissey JP, McGreevy MM: The fates of applicants denied admission to state mental hospitals: some unexamined consequences of deinstitutionalization in the U.S.A. Paper presented at the meeting of the International Sociological Association, Mexico City, August 1982

135. Pepper B, Ryglewicz H: Testimony for the neglected: the mentally ill in the post-deinstitutionalized age. Am J Orthopsychiatry 52:388–392, 1982

136. Sullivan R: Hospital forced to oust patients with psychoses. The New York Times, 8 November 1979, p B3

137. Sullivan R: Hospitals will gain by cutting bed use. The New York Times, 31 December 1979, p A1

138. James JF: Principles in developing a community support system. Hosp Community Psychiatry 29:34–35, 1978

139. Levine IS: Service programs for the homeless mentally ill, in The Homeless Mentally Ill: A Task Force Report of the American Psychiatric Association. Edited by Lamb HR. Washington, DC, American Psychiatric Association, 1984

140. Schwartz T: Homeless given help on streets. The New York Times, 1 September 1979, pp 21–22

141. Bachrach LL: Conference reports: research on services for the homeless mentally ill. Hosp Community Psychiatry 35:910–913, 1984

142. Rule S: Needs of homeless bring forth caring volunteers. The New York Times, 8 April 1984, p 54

143. Rubenstein C: Skid row pays tribute to residents, friends who have died. Oregonian [Portland], 30 March 1984, p B1

144. Chase A: St. Francis House is symbol of renewal for homeless. The Washington Post, 5 May 1984, p B6

145. Gray P: A hot meal for those whose home is on the street. Maryland Today (University of Maryland, Adelphi), March 1984, p 9

146. Schanberg SH: The expendable people. The New York Times, 15 December 1981, p A31

147. Zoerhide JS: Everyone gains as Baltimore church feeds the hungry. Unitarian Universalist World, 15 May 1984, pp 1, 10

148. No Place Like Home. Aired on the State Line Series, Maryland Public Television, Channel 22, Annapolis, 25 December 1983

CHAPTER 5

Innovative Treatment and Rehabilitation Techniques for the Chronic Mentally Ill

ROBERT P. LIBERMAN, M.D.
CATHERINE C. PHIPPS, M.S.

Effective treatment for acute episodes of major mental disorders is now available for most patients. Usually within a relatively brief, intensive treatment period of weeks to months, the positive symptoms of schizophrenic, affective, anxiety, and substance abuse disorders can be significantly ameliorated with appropriate drugs and milieu therapy. Acute treatment can be effectively delivered in outpatient, day hospital, and inpatient settings. Unfortunately, treatment of acute episodes, while enormously helpful, does not provide for the comprehensive needs of many mental patients. Just as with most medical disorders, such as arteriosclerotic heart disease, hypertension, kidney and liver diseases, diabetes, arthritis, headaches, and multiple sclerosis, most mental disorders are chronic in course with cyclical remissions and exacerbations and long periods of impairment; thus, long-term treatment and rehabilitation strategies are required. Treatment services offered to patients for acute and intermittent relapses and exacerbations fail to meet their long-term needs for adaptation, restoration of function, and maintenance of well-being.

We will define long-term treatment as rehabilitation since there is a comparable rehabilitation approach to that for medically ill patients. Just as cardiac rehabilitation begins after the patient with the myocardial infarct leaves the intensive coronary care unit, and physical therapy begins after the patient with an amputated limb leaves the surgical suite, rehabilitation of the patient with schizophrenia or bipolar disorder begins after antipsychotic medications bring delusions, hallucinations, incoherence, and agitation into relative remission or stabilization. Even for those patients who do not respond well to acute treatment interventions—and it can be estimated that as many as 20 percent of schizophrenics are refractory to short-term pharmacotherapy—long-term psychiatric rehabilitation is still indicated. What cannot be accomplished in a hurry can often be dealt with over a longer period of consistent and systematic intervention (1).

Psychiatric rehabilitation has five major goals (2):

1. To ameliorate the positive symptoms of a disorder that do not remit with brief treatment.
2. To maintain the gains made by the patient during acute treatment and to prevent or delay the reemergence of symptoms over the long haul.
3. To assist the patient in managing and reducing the negative or deficit symptoms of major mental disorders that pose a largely unanswered challenge to the pharmacopeia; for example, social withdrawal, apathy, anergy, slovenliness, and anhedonia do not respond as well to neuroleptic drugs as do the positive symptoms of schizophrenia.
4. To inculcate or restore social and living skills which may never have been learned or which may have atrophied during periods of illness and hospitalization.
5. To modify the patient's social environment toward more supportive and less stressful qualities.

Before reviewing some new techniques in psychiatric rehabilitation of chronic mental patients, a short detour around the conceptual landscape of chronic mental disorders will help point us in directions for effective interventions.

CHRONIC MENTAL DISORDER IN BIOSOCIAL-BEHAVIORAL PERSPECTIVE

There is a growing consensus that schizophrenia and other major mental disorders can be understood—in terms of etiology and course—as being determined by biobehavioral vulnerability, environmental stressors and supports, and personal coping and competence. The symptoms and impairments that constitute the chronic mental disorders can be viewed as being in equilibrium with biological and environmental determinants. The appearance or increase in characteristic symptoms of a severe mental disorder may occur in a susceptible individual when:

1. the underlying biological susceptibility or vulnerability increases, either through natural internal cycles or through drug and alcohol abuse;
2. stressful life events overwhelm the individual's coping skills in social and instrumental roles;
3. the individual cannot cope with demands and tensions of everyday life because social problem-solving skills either have never been learned, or, if the individual previously had them in his/her repertoire, they have withered as a result of disuse, reinforcement of the sick role, or loss of motivation;
4. the individual's social support network weakens or diminishes.

Psychotropic medication reduces a person's vulnerability to relapse and protects the person from the stressful impact of life events and tension-filled family relationships (3–5); however, the modulation of biologic vulnerability by medication cannot fully protect a vulnerable individual from relapse due to stressors, loss of social support, or diminution in problem-solving skills. Even with reliable ingestion of neuroleptics about 40 percent of newly discharged schizophrenic patients relapse within a year (6). From this vantage point, an increase or reappearance of symptoms in a person vulnerable to a major mental disorder is an outcome of the balance or interaction between the number of life stressors and the problem-solving capacities of the individual and his/her support network (7).

A somewhat simplified interactive model of schizophrenic symptom formation and impairments in role functioning is presented in Figure 1. Schizophrenia is chosen as the illustrative disorder because it comprises the majority of individuals termed chronically mentally ill; however, the model would be compatible with most other major mental disorders as well. The model includes personal and environmental factors—social competence and social supports, respectively, that serve to protect an individual from relapse; psychobiologic vulnerability factors; and external stressors. Through an interactional process, these variables result in the florid symptoms and associated disabilities of schizophrenia.

Social stressors include life events as well as exposure to critical and emotionally overinvolved family members. Loss or estrangement of friends, relatives, neighbors, co-workers, and help-givers all reduce the supportiveness of the social network. The effects of social stressors and social network variables are assumed to interact; for example, the death of a loved one may be compounded by the lack of other social support or may be minimized by the presence of other supportive figures. Vulnerable individuals may experience stress from even minor, everyday events and interactions such as shopping, preparing a meal, or casually talking with

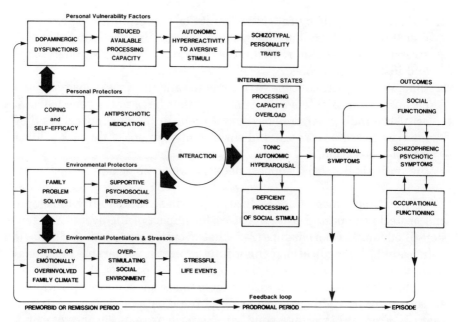

Figure 1. A simplified interactive model of schizophrenic symptoms formation and impairments in role functioning.

a relative. These stressors challenge underdeveloped or underused life skills. Alternatively, social competence may serve as a protective factor against symptoms and functional impairments as well.

Enduring, trait-like characteristics of an individual reflect vulnerability and biologic diathesis to schizophrenia. Presumed central nervous system traits may be manifested by dysfunctions in information processing and arousal. These dysfunctions may be relatively permanent but latent, becoming detectable only when the individual is unduly stressed. In other cases, the underlying vulnerability, genetic loading, and psychologic dysfunctions may be so great that even minor life events or small losses of social support may tip the balance into psychosis. In either case, the preexisting vulnerability makes the individual susceptible to symptom formation.

In summary, a vulnerability–stress interactive model of the formation of schizophrenic symptoms consists of noxious social events that combine with preexisting vulnerability to produce intermediate states of sensory overload, hyperarousal, and impaired processing of social stimuli (8). These intermediate states and their behavioral concomitants generate even more stressors, leading to the appearance of schizophrenic symptoms and impaired functioning. The model suggests points of entry for treatment intervention. Strategies for drug treatment, for example, might include increased dosages or intermittent prescription of neuroleptics timed to coincide with periods of increased stress or early warning signals of symptom exacerbation. Psychosocial therapies might be designed to affect those socioenvironmental stressors, personal coping skills, and social support linkages implicated in the pathogenesis of symptom formation.

In the lexicon of the rehabilitation practitioner are terms such as impairment, disability, and handicap. In major mental disorders, it is presumed that underlying biologic vulnerability combined with inadequate protection from an individual's social competence and social support network lead to abnormalities in central nervous system function that appear as *impairments* in cognitive information processing, psychobiologic states, and symptom formation. In turn, these psychobiologic *impairments* lead to *disabilities* in the affected person's social and occupational functioning; for example, the individual may withdraw from friends and family and may not be able to continue working because of distractibility, loss of both concentration and interest in the job, and the intrusion of delusions and hallucinations. Finally, if these disabilities persist and there is no accommodation by the person's social and vocational environments, *handicaps* develop. For example, if the family and work systems are mystified by the person's disabilities, do not view them as part of a bona fide illness, and are unyielding in their expectations for normal social and job performance, it is likely that the disabled person will be *handicapped* in his or her roles as a participating family member and worker.

Rehabilitation and treatment strategies can be directed at one or more of these points in the chain that lead to a handicap. Psychotropic medication, rationally prescribed and reliably used, can reduce *impairments*. Drugs such as lithium and the neuroleptics have potent effects on the positive symptoms of severe mental disorders. They also improve cognitive processes, attentional and arousal mechanisms, and learning capacities. Training of social and vocational skills can remediate a patient's *disabilities*. Supportive home and work environments that make allowances for the individual's impairments and disabilities and actively compensate for them can prevent or reverse *handicaps*. For example, a sheltered workshop or transitional employment program that includes initially lowered and then gradually increasing expectations of performance combined with supportiveness from supervisors and counselors can enable even a markedly disabled person with a mental disorder to function in the worker role. Similarly, family therapy can educate relatives about mental disorder, helping them to at least temporarily lower their expectations of the patient's sociability and functioning. The family system can acquire coping skills to more flexibly respond to the patient's realistic needs and disabilities, which enables the patient to sustain respect and integrity as a family member.

In the next sections of this chapter, we delineate some innovative treatment and rehabilitation strategies and techniques that have shown promise in reducing *impairments*, *disabilities*, and *handicaps*. With chronic mental disorders that produce severe impairments, complex disabilities, and handicaps, it is understandable that a wide range of interventions are necessary to achieve rehabilitation goals. Medication alone is rarely sufficient, and psychosocial methods have little chance of success if isolated from the judicious use of psychotropic drugs. It is almost a truism among experienced clinicians that pharmacotherapy and psychosocial therapy should play supplementary and not competing roles in the comprehensive management of schizophrenic patients. Most experienced clinicians view neuroleptic therapy as accomplishing reconstitutive and prophylactic goals. In ameliorating the cognitive disorganization and disabling symptoms of psychosis, drugs enable the patient to make effective contact with the environment and engage in a therapeutic alliance with a therapist or psychosocial program. Continuity of care that integrates both maintenance medication and pursuit of personal, social, and instrumental role goals has the best chance of restoring the individual with schizophrenia to a functional existence and reasonable quality of life.

INNOVATIONS IN PHARMACOTHERAPY

Perhaps the most obvious implication for intervention from the multitiered model of mental disorder depicted above is the value of somatic therapies for reducing a genetically susceptible individual's biologic vulnerability to the emergence of signs and symptoms of mental illness. Unfortunately, there have been few new advances, beyond the refinement of drug classes to alter side effect profiles, since the development of psychotropic drugs for psychosis, mania, depression, and anxiety in the 1950s and 1960s. The second and third generation of antidepressant and antipsychotic drugs have not been found to offer significantly greater therapeutic benefits, and no major new drug discoveries appear to be on the horizon. Drugs, instead, have served as neuropharmacologic probes to help neuroscientists better understand the functioning of normal and deviant central nervous systems.

Some modest innovations in psychopharmacotherapy have been reported. For example, carbamazepine (Tegretol), which was originally used as an anticonvulsant, has been shown to be effective in patients with lithium-resistant mania and perhaps also for patients experiencing depression. Lithium, when added to an antidepressant, appears to augment the therapeutic effect of the antidepressant and can help patients who are refractory to the antidepressant alone. Antidepressants have recently been documented as helpful in controlling and preventing panic episodes and in the overall treatment of bulimia.

There is a growing recognition of the problems of nonadherence to maintenance neuroleptic and lithium medication (9), which has led to the development and empirical testing of educational strategies for improving patients' understanding and acceptance of long-term medication for schizophrenia and bipolar disorder (10–11). Another important innovation has been the development of new strategies for neuroleptic pharmacotherapy of schizophrenia that lessen overall exposure to the drugs and may reduce toxic and potentially irreversible effects of these agents while sustaining their therapeutic benefits.

The 1978 American Psychiatric Association (APA) publication *The Chronic Mental Patient* highlights the importance of aggressive monitoring and compliance with neuroleptic drug regimens in the community adaptation of schizophrenics (9). However, recent research has cast doubt on the critical importance of the standard recommended doses of maintenance medication in preventing relapse. It has become increasingly clear that neuroleptics do not prevent, but at best only delay, relapse. One multihospital, well-controlled study comparing oral and injectable depot fluphenazine found that the relapse rates were equal—about 40 percent by the end of the first year (6). Thus, the long-acting depot injections of Prolixin Decanoate, which assured reliable administration, did not result in a lower rate of relapse than the orally administered form of the drug. It is now being suggested that perhaps early and prodromal signs of relapse occur *before* a schizophrenic patient discontinues his or her medication and that medication noncompliance may be a consequence rather than a cause of some relapses.

While neuroleptic drugs are clearly efficacious for the schizophrenic—as lithium and antidepressants are for those suffering from affective disorders—it is also likely that most patients are receiving doses much higher than they need, thereby raising the risk/benefit ratio. It has become increasingly clear that neuroleptic drugs, and to a lesser extent lithium and antidepressants, produce serious side effects that compromise their value to an already impaired individual. For example, the disabling negative symptoms of schizophrenia, such as affective blunting and flatness, anhedonia, listlessness, apathy, and social withdrawal, are worsened by such neuroleptic-induced side effects as akinesia, akathisia, sedation, and possibly depression. Currently used doses of neuroleptics may actually be "poisoning" many of our schizophrenic patients by increasing the negative symptoms of their disorder (12). The most dreaded of the neuroleptic side effects, irreversible tardive dyskinesia, has been found in 12 percent of individuals at the end of four years of cumulative neuroleptic drug exposure (13).

The task of the prescribing psychiatrist is to provide the benefits of neuroleptic drug treatment while minimizing the risk of tardive dyskinesia and the severity of other side effects such as akinesia that further impair performance of patients. Alternative drug strategies have been proposed that reduce the overall cumulative dose of a drug. One such dosage strategy uses a substantially lower amount of neuroleptic than has ordinarily been thought to be effective for maintaining patients in symptomatic remission. In an ongoing study by Marder and his colleagues (12), 5 mg of long-acting fluphenazine has been found as effective as 25 mg for preventing relapse and has been associated with significantly fewer side effects. Patients on the lower dose report significantly less subjective dysphoria and distress. Using an even lower maintenance dose of fluphenazine, Kane and his colleagues (14) reported higher rates of symptom exacerbation in the low-dose group but much less tardive dyskinesia. Furthermore, patients treated with the very low dose of drug who did relapse were able to return to acceptable levels of functioning quickly after relatively brief hospitalizations or temporary increases in their drug dose. Even for those patients receiving low-dose therapy who relapsed, their families rated them significantly more favorably in terms of social performance.

A second novel drug reduction treatment strategy is "targeted" or "intermittent" medication (15, 16). This strategy is based on the view that patients do not require antipsychotic medication at all times but only during periods of symptom exacerbation or incipient relapse. Without continuous protection from medication, patients on targeted or intermittent drugs must be in close contact with and collaborating positively with physicians and relatives so that early signs of symptoms worsening can be detected and drug treatment rapidly introduced. In addition, it is advisable that patients who are chosen for this type of drug strategy are able to acknowledge their illness and to identify early warning signals of relapse and are willing to contact their responsible physician or treatment team when symptoms begin to intrude. Studies that are still in progress have yielded preliminary data that suggest that intermittent and targeted neuroleptic therapy can successfully prevent hospitalization with less psychopathology and much lower cumulative doses of medication.

EFFECTIVE PSYCHOSOCIAL PROGRAMS FOR THE CHRONIC MENTALLY ILL

In APA's *The Chronic Mental Patient,* published in 1978, two chapters were devoted to describing effective programs of care. The paucity of well-controlled, scientifically respectable research on effective programs was decried; only three comprehensive programs were described as having reliable and valid data supporting their efficacy. These programs were: 1) the "Social Learning Program," a behaviorally based, highly structured residential program with declining-contact community aftercare. This program employed educational, problem-solving, and skills training integrated with ongoing assessment systems and reinforcement contingencies (1); 2) The Training in Community Living Program (TCL), in which patients received at-home assistance and training in meeting community living needs through intensive care management services (17); and 3) the "Fountain House" social rehabilitation program, which used self-help social clubs and transitional and supportive residential and employment opportunities (18).

We followed up the 1978 APA report with a literature review from 1978–1984, searching for empirically validated studies of psychosocial treatment and rehabilitation programs for chronic mental patients. To ensure that only carefully peer-reviewed studies would be included, we limited our search to 12 highly esteemed psychiatric and psychologic journals that are well known for the thorough, scientific criteria used by their editorial boards in accepting articles for publication. These journals included the *Journal of Consulting and Clinical Psychology, American Psychologist, Journal of Applied Behavior Analysis, Behavior Therapy, Archives of General Psychiatry, American Journal of Psychiatry, Psychiatry Research, British Journal of Psychiatry, Psychological Medicine, Psychological Bulletin, Behaviour Research and Therapy,* and the *Schizophrenia Bulletin.* Over the five and one-half year screening period, only nine articles were found in these journals that reported effective psychosocial treatments for the chronic mentally ill, again highlighting the deplorable lack of clinical research in this area.

Two of the nine articles that we found presented further data attesting to the effectivness of the TCL and Fountain House programs. Stein and Test (19) documented that their TCL program was an effective alternative to hospitalization. One hundred and thirty chronic mental patients were randomly assigned to hospital-based or community-based treatment for 14 months. Hospitalized patients were treated as inpatients for as long as necessary to bring symptoms into reasonable remission and then were linked with community agencies for aftercare. Experimental patients did not enter the hospital; instead they received services from the TCL program for 14 months and then were integrated into existing community programs. Almost all of the experimental group maintained community tenure for the 14 months in which they received TCL services with no greater symptoms or impairments than the hospitalized patients. In addition, patients in the TCL group scored higher on measures of self-esteem and personal satisfaction with life and worked more than those patients who were initially hospitalized. Follow-up results indicated that when patients were weaned from the TCL program, their superior personal and vocational status waned and their use of the hospital increased. In subsequent publications and presentations, the developers of the TCL program had advocated continuing and indefinite use of intensive care management services for maintaining clinical and community adjustment.

Two studies were conducted at Fountain House (20) that examined the influence of psychiatric rehabilitation services on rehospitalization rates. The first study was begun in 1959 and utilized 252 Fountain House members and 81 control subjects who were followed for nine years. Results revealed that the Fountain House members had significantly lower rehospitalization rates for the first five years in the study, spending twice as long in the community before needing rehospitalization and 40 percent fewer days in the hospital than control subjects. The second study, a replication of the first, began in 1964 with 40 Fountain House members and 34 controls who were followed for five years. Again it was found that the Fountain House members had significantly lower rehospitalization rates for the first two years of the study, remaining in the community almost three times longer than control subjects.

A third comprehensive treatment and rehabilitation program, Soteria House, employed intensive and humanistically oriented psychotherapy and minimal medication with first or second episode, young adult psychotics. The comparison group, which was not randomly selected, received conventional psychiatric services through the local community mental health center. Results were mixed inasmuch as most measures of clinical status did not differentiate the treatment conditions, although independent living rates were higher and overall medication use lower for the Soteria House patients than for those who received customary care. While the Soteria House was staffed with largely nonprofessional therapists, this cost savings was mitigated by much longer stays in the House than the hospitalization periods for the comparison sample (21).

Of the four comprehensive treatment and rehabilitation programs that have received empirical validation of their effectiveness over the past 15 years, only two have been replicated in a number of new locales—

Fountain House and TCL. One additional efficacious program not previously described, the Community Lodge approach to transitional employment and living of Fairweather and his associates (22), was systematically disseminated to and adopted by a large number of other agencies. However, when one surveys the current state of services for the chronically mentally ill, there is too little evidence of the impact of these model programs. While there are many sociopolitical, fiscal, and bureaucratic reasons for the failure of greater penetration by sound, demonstrably effective programs (22–24), one obstacle may lie in their very comprehensiveness and distinctiveness.

While it has been pointed out that comprehensiveness of services for the many needs of chronic mental patients distinguishes model programs (25), this very asset can also be a liability in efforts to "transport" such programs to new settings. Because of a variety of local constraints in financing, personnel practices, resources, patient populations, and organizational structures, it may be very difficult to implant a complex, many-faceted program in places distant from its home turf. Some programs have surmounted these obstacles; for example, the Community Lodge program of Fairweather and his colleagues; the Fountain House psychosocial club program; and the Training in Community Living program of Stein and Test have all been widely adopted by other sites. However, it has taken very special dissemination efforts to promote this level of adoption; for example, activities in which potential adoptees can visit and receive training in a host-demonstration program during extended periods were required.

In contrast to those innovations that require minimal change in current practices for adoption by individual service providers—such as office-based behavior therapy techniques and new psychotropic drugs—comprehensive psychosocial programs have unique requirements for dissemination, if their integrity is to be maintained (26). If an organization wishes to adopt a comprehensive program, decision makers must be involved at several levels. In addition to training in new psychosocial technologies, major changes in the roles of service providers, organizational structures, and operating principles are required. Consequently, the time frame is lengthy between development and widespread dissemination for such programs, involving two decades in the case of the Teaching-Family program for delinquent adolescents and the Community Lodge program for adult mental patients. Not only are detailed written and audiovisual training materials necessary, but available host-demonstration programs and/or a cadre of knowledgeable personnel are needed to provide direct, hands-on training in the new technologies over extended time periods. Thus, even though firm plans to implement the Social Learning Program of Paul and his associates (26) have been made by over 20 facilities or departments in 13 states and two Canadian provinces, their clinical research group has had to temporarily discourage implementations in all but two sites. This is because extensive training materials for the assessment system that is needed to support the treatment program and insure its integrity must first be completed for efficient widespread dissemination.

An alternative strategy for transferring effective rehabilitation technology to new locales may be found in the concept of "modules." A module, in treatment and rehabilitation terms, is a relatively discrete, circumscribed, and delimited program element or intervention that serves specific functions, aims at limited goals, works with well-defined populations, can be easily learned by neophyte staff, and requires relatively little in the way of social and environmental support. Modules that are validated for their impact on a limited set of outcome criteria can survive in hostile institutional and agency climates because they do not challenge or contradict established traditions and ideologies. Modules or elements, newly designed or adapted from larger comprehensive programs, usually cost very little to adopt in terms of time, money, effort, and special personnel requirements.

Thus, modules might be more rapidly disseminated into mental health and rehabilitation services since they do not require major changes in the roles of service providers or organizational structures of existing agencies. They may also be adopted by individual service providers without requiring organizational decisions, which are more subject to complex political factors (24, 26). The modular approach might, therefore, lead to more rapid incremental improvements in existing services without the extended time lags of comprehensive programs. Moreover, well-tested modules could easily be incorporated within the curriculum of broader and more comprehensive programs for chronic mental patients.

Modules can be designed to fit the special needs of a wide variety of patients. If new patient characteristics arise that are incongruent with an existing module, a new module can be quickly fabricated. Modules can be designed for skill building at various levels of baseline, entry-level functioning of patients or can be organized as an environmental prosthesis to simply maintain and support a patient's current level of functioning. Modules can be collectively organized to construct a comprehensive program that is mandated to meet the needs of a designated catchment area and spectrum of patients. Since priorities within a mental health system often change, modules can be adapted to meet these shifting priorities. For example, at the West Los Angeles VA Medical Center, social skills training modules were quickly revised from intensive and long-term use with a small number of patients to short-term use with a very large number of referred patients when turnover and utilization priorities changed at the Medical Center.

In the remainder of this chapter, we demonstrate the modular approach to treatment and rehabilitation of the chronic mental patient, primarily through illustrations of three modules or elements that aim at building social, vocational, and living skills. A fourth example will come from our efforts to construct a resource book for professionals in rehabilitation and mental health that consists of program elements that have been found to be effective and useful and which we have "modularized" through operational descriptions.

Training Social and Living Skills

Social skills training has proven to be an effective way of increasing the social competence of chronic mental patients (27, 28). There are three sources of empirical data that recommend social skills training as a means for improving patients' competence and ability to cope with stressors. Many studies have highlighted the importance of premorbid and postmorbid social competence as a predictor of outcome in major psychiatric disorders (29–33). This suggests that social skills training might improve long-term prognosis by upgrading the postmorbid social competence of chronic patients. Second, the magnitude of deficits in social and living skills has been well documented in chronic psychiatric patients. For example, in one study, major functional deficits in social and personal areas were found in over 50 percent of a sample of chronic psychiatric patients (32). A multihospital study of schizophrenic patients placed in foster homes after relatively brief hospitalizations found that relapse rates at one year after discharge were significantly higher among those patients who had prerelease deficiencies in social skills (33). In another large-scale study in which depressed and normal patients were compared, social introversion and interpersonal dependency were the most significant premorbid personal characteristics discriminating the patient sample (30).

Third, certain types of family interaction patterns have been implicated in the course of schizophrenia and depression (4, 34). Four studies conducted in London and Los Angeles over a 10-year period have shown that criticism and emotional overinvolvement by relatives significantly increase the probability of relapse. This suggests that improving the problem-solving and communication skills of family members, as well as the social and independent living skills of patients, might have a beneficial impact on relapse, family burden, and social adjustment.

In the aforementioned literature search, four of the nine publications describing efficacious programs were modules for training social and living skills (35–38). The learning of social and living skills is usually facilitated by the concurrent administration of appropriate types and doses of psychotropic drugs.

Social skills training utilizes procedures based on principles of human learning to train specific interpersonal skills and to promote the generalization and maintenance of these skills. The procedures that have been developed to train interpersonal skills have been empirically tested and "packaged" for ready access by practitioners.

While many psychosocial programs bill themselves as offering social skills training, it is important to distinguish between nonspecific group activities that engage patients in "socialization" and methods that deliberately and systematically utilize behavioral learning techniques in a structured approach to skills building. While socialization activities can lead to acquisition of skills through incidental learning during spontaneous social interactions, they do not harness social learning and reinforcement techniques that may be required to promote the acquisition, generalization, and durability of skills needed in interpersonal situations (39).

The learning disabilities experienced by many chronic psychiatric patients require the use of highly directive behavioral techniques for training social skills. For example, most chronic patients have attentional and information-processing deficits. They show hyperarousal or underarousal in psychophysiologic testing, and they experience overstimulation from emotional stressors or even from therapy sessions that are not carefully structured and modulated. Chronic patients often fail to be motivated by the customary forms of social and tangible rewards available in traditional therapy. In addition, they generally lack conversational ability, a basic building block for social competence. Schizophrenics, in particular, are deficient in social perception and have difficulty generating alternatives for coping with everyday problems such as missing a bus, making an appointment, or getting help with bothersome drug side effects. Patients tend to make less eye contact, have more verbal dysfluencies, and use less vocal intonation, all of which may impair social learning.

It is important to tailor social skills training procedures to the needs of the individual patient, as patients present different constellations of social abilities and deficiencies. Several training models are presently available to the clinician. Longest in use is a treatment package for training skills that includes specific, goal-oriented instructions to the patient, the therapist modeling appropriate use of the skills, the patient role-playing interpersonal situations, and the therapist reinforcing and providing corrective feedback to the patient. Recently, training within an information-processing framework has been shown to be effective for those patients capable of learning problem-solving strategies (40). Patients are taught to improve their perception of information in immediate interpersonal situations, process that information to choose a response, and send a response back to the other person. However, both of these approaches are ineffective for those patients with severe attentional deficiencies. A model using attention-focusing procedures based on stimulus control technology, which simplifies the learning of complex skills, has been effective in training conversational skills in some seriously regressed, chronic psychiatric patients (41).

A basic social skills training module, termed training in personal effectiveness (39), was validated as effective with a wide range of chronic mental patients in a typical community mental health center (42). It was then "packaged" for dissemination by including an instructional manual, explicit directions for acquiring the relevant therapy skills through learning exercises, and a demonstration film. Staff members from 40 community mental health centers in a wide range of rural and urban locales throughout the United States participated in a training process that began with a two-day workshop featuring live demonstrations, role playing, and a "contract" with staff members who agreed to continue with further inservice training. Peer tutors were utilized for subsequent training exercises, and each mental health center chose an internal coordinator who "championed" the implementation of the module.

Statistically significant increases were found in the participating staff members' knowledge of, attitudes toward, and utilization of the social skills training module. In 61 percent of the mental health centers, a substantial contingent of staff members reported implementing regularly scheduled social skills training in group and individual therapy (43).

Behavioral Family Management

Employing the same learning principles and techniques that are integral to social skills training, a three-pronged module was developed for enhancing the communication and problem-solving skills of families containing a schizophrenic member (44). Despite the development of community mental health programs and the widespread use of neuroleptic drugs, families continue to serve as the principal caregivers for schizophrenic patients. While the burden of providing emotional, social, and instrumental supports for schizophrenics has always fallen mainly on the patients' relatives, this burden has become even greater since the deinstitutionalization movement of the past 20 years. Based upon intensive interviews with 80 relatives of schizophrenics, a report titled *Schizo-phrenia at Home*, which summarized the problems described by the relatives, was issued (45). Problems fell into three major categories: 1) distress caused by the patients' symptomatic and socially impaired behavior; 2) anxiety and "burnout" experiences by the relatives; and 3) disturbances in the relatives' own social network.

From the point of view of relatives, schizophrenic family members living at home display two types of behavior that are distressing and difficult to cope with. Social withdrawal and solitary patterns, on the one hand, and aggressive, bizarre, and disruptive behavior, on the other, are found in varying degrees at different points in time during the course of the illness. Social isolation, to the point of rarely exchanging conversation, is the more common pattern; it generates helpless frustration in relatives whose sustained social support for such patients requires a modicum of responsiveness. Another facet of isolated behavior is the apathy and indolence of the chronic schizophrenic, which galls relatives who view the patients as physically able and do not understand such absence of constructive activity.

Relatives speak of being "constantly on a knife edge," "living on your nerves," or "feeling in constant dread of relapse and flare-ups of symptoms." Guilt, exhaustion, depression, anxiety, and anger are frequent experiences of relatives that, in combination with the patients' deviance, do much to explain the high "expressed emotion" in families—a factor that has been found to predict relapse (4, 34, 46, 47). Expressed emotion, consisting of criticism, hostility, and emotional overinvolvement, is an understandable reaction of concerned family members who are at a loss to know how to help their schizophrenic relatives. Overinvolvement can lead a family giving up its attachments to the outside community and to spending inordinate amounts of time at home with the patient. Criticism and hostility can lead to rejection of the patient, and, ultimately, to a breach of the relationship.

The behavioral family management module was designed for use with individual families and with multiple family groups and can be adapted for use with families of patients with other major mental disorders. It has been offered less intensively over nine weekly, two-hour sessions or, for more definitive skill-building, during a two-year period (weekly sessions for three months; biweekly sessions for six months; then monthly maintenance sessions). In three empirical evaluations and controlled studies, it has been shown to reduce family tensions, conflicts, and expressed emotion, markedly reduce relapse rates and rehospitalization, enhance problem-solving and coping, improve social adjustment of patients, and lessen family burden (48, 49). Cost-effectiveness analysis indicated that a home-based version of behavioral family management was much more effective and less costly than comparable clinic-based treatment of individuals. Data from a controlled clinical trial comparing behavioral family therapy with individual therapy are given in Table 1.

The three facets of behavioral family management include education about schizophrenia and its treatment, training in communication skills, and training in a stepwise and systematic problem-solving process. The initial sessions are used to educate relatives and patients about schizophrenia, its causes, course, and management. Detailed information is presented, and patients and their families are invited to discuss their own experiences and to express their own feelings and concerns. These sessions function to relieve some of the guilt, confusion, and helplessness experienced by family members, as well as to foster realistic expectations

Table 1. Outcomes of Behavioral Family Management and Individual Therapy for Schizophrenics ($N = 18$ in each group)

	Family Rx	Individual Rx
Relapses (no. of patients)		
Nine months**	1	8
Two years**	2	15
Target symptom ratings (average score)		
Nine months**	2.25	4.10
Two years**	2.55	4.75
Symptom remission (no. of patients)		
Nine months*	10	4
Two years**	12	4
Time spent in rehospitalizations (average no. of days)		
Nine months	0.83	8.39
Two years	1.8	11.3
No. of patients readmitted to hospital		
Nine months*	2	9
Two years*	4	10
Household tasks (improvement)**	0.36	−0.09
Work or study (improvement)*	0.36	−0.14
Relationships outside (improvement)**	0.65	0.09
Cost per unit of effectiveness	$2,220	$5,167

Note. Patients in both psychosocial treatment conditions received optimal neuroleptic drug therapy. * $p < .05$. ** $f < .01$.

about treatment outcome and to emphasize the importance of continued maintenance medication. The impact of schizophrenia upon each family member and problems of management are discussed. The educational seminars are presented in a semididactic style with visual aids and written materials. The patient is encouraged to take the role of "expert" and to describe his or her experiences to the family.

Following these information-giving sessions, the objective is to provide training in communication and problem-solving skills. Each session is devoted to identification of problems facing the entire family, with training in relevant communication skills. The therapist demonstrates effective and ineffective communication skills in brief role plays. This is followed by guided practice with feedback to teach four types of communication:

1. Expressing positive feelings and giving positive feedback.
2. Making requests of others; expressing expectations and setting rules.
3. Using active listening skills to learn the needs and emotions of others.
4. Expressing directly negative emotions and feelings of anger and disapproval.

The initial phase of enhancing communication skills of family members focuses on the expression of positive feelings through prompting mutually rewarding behavior and empathic listening. The aim of the early stage of family therapy is to create a warm milieu where family members are able to recognize and reinforce specific positive behavior in one another. In addition, they learn to identify areas of specific behavior they would like others to change, as well as to make appropriate requests for such changes. Finally, they develop the ability to sit down and discuss problems in an emphatic, nonjudgmental manner. Expression of strong negative feelings is taken up after positive communication and interaction have been established. Communication skills are important precursors to successful problem-solving discussions.

Once families have developed adequate communication skills, they are then in a position to learn improved problem-solving methods. The ability to specify a problem and to discuss it in detail can only be carried out by families that have competent communication skills. Patients and their families are taught to do the following:

1. Pinpoint and specify problems in living.
2. Develop several options or alternative responses.
3. Evaluate each option in terms of its possible consequences.
4. Choose option(s) that maximize(s) satisfaction and seem(s) reasonable.

5. Plan how to implement that option (or those options) as a family.
6. Provide mutual support in the implementation.
7. Review the problem after the selected option has been implemented.

These problem-solving steps are repeatedly used to analyze and focus on a wide range of family problems, especially those that are associated with tension and conflict. The repetitive practice of problem solving, together with repeated practice of the four basic communication skills, is aimed at inculcating durable and general problem-solving strategies.

Families are provided with sheets that outline the steps, with spaces for completion of problem solving. Particular importance is attached to the detailed planning of the problem solution, with all anticipated difficulties discussed fully. Each family member takes a turn at chairing the family problem-solving sessions and recording details of the problem, all suggested solutions, and step-by-step plans to carry out the chosen "best" solution. A folder is kept by each family in which members file all problem-solving records. This folder is kept in an accessible place in each home so that any family member may refer to it at any time. Sometimes problem-solving plans may be displayed on the family notice board or on the refrigerator door to remind family members of the tasks they have agreed to undertake to assist with the problems.

In addition to the structured problem-solving approach, families are trained in the use of a range of behavioral strategies for dealing with specific problems that arise. These may include contingency contracting for parental discord, token economy programs for enhancing constructive daily activity, social skills training for interpersonal inadequacy, or behavioral management strategies for anxiety and depression. In these instances, all family members are usually involved in the execution of the specific strategy.

Behavioral family management has begun to be packaged and disseminated. A manual has been written for prospective therapists, and a videotape for training workshops has been produced. Workshops are being designed to engage the active participation in a learning mode of multidisciplinary workers in rehabilitation and mental health. The National Institute of Mental Health (NIMH) has sponsored a multicenter collaborative research project to replicate and extend the methods, results, and implications of the original studies on behavioral family management. Comparisons will be made with a briefer and less intensive and structured crisis intervention approach to family management. In addition, the two psychosocial treatments will be factored with three medication conditions—intermittent targeted drug, continuous low-dose drug, and continuous standard-dose drug. Within another three years, it will be possible to determine the degree to which behavioral family measurement can be feasibly transferred to other sites and therapists.

Job Finding Club

The reciprocal relatonship between work and health is sewn into the fabric of our lives. Unless accidents or illness produce disabilities, most people can expect to work for 40 to 45 years. Work provides money for survival and adds quality to life. Work provides status; respect from self and others; a functional role in an organization, community, and society; and socialization and friends. When, for structural reasons during economic downturns, unemployment rates zoom upward, the incidence of mental disorders and rate of psychiatric hospitalization also rise (50). Clinically oriented studies have found correlations between unemployment and suicide rates, depressed mood, and other physical and psychologic symptoms (51). In the Training in Community Living program described above, chronic psychiatric patients were placed in sheltered workshops, in regular jobs, and in transitional volunteer jobs with charitable agencies. From the point of view of work, this community-based program produced twice as much work capacity as gauged by earnings as did a standard state hospital treatment. In addition, those patients who were actively involved in sheltered or competitive employment were the least likely to relapse and return to the hospital (52).

Work is perceived as important by individuals suffering from major mental disorders. In a survey of 500 chronic mental patients residing in Los Angeles board-and-care homes, Lehman et al. (53) found that lack of work was one of the greatest complaints related to poor quality of life. Even chronically impaired patients supported by Social Security pensions had not relinquished their aspirations for a job—their dissatisfication with unemployment and leisure time was significantly greater than a cross-section of the normal population. Despite these aspirations, unemployment has been reported to be as high as 70 percent in the chronically mentally disabled (54).

Another way to appreciate the functional connection between psychopathology and work is to view it from the vantage point of individuals who have mental illnesses and who are working. For example, one such individual described the impact of work on his symptoms in the following manner: "Work helps me organize my thoughts, makes me feel less crazy. It keeps me busy so I don't get bored, then depressed. I think better and concentrate more when I'm not depressed. When I'm bored, my thoughts go wild" (55). Being able to work may also compensate for the social stigma attached to the mentally ill. In our society, which places such a high premium on work, family members and friends often tolerate an individual's deviant behavior in direct proportion to his ability to perform in the world of work.

There is no denying that psychiatric patients often have difficulty locating employment. Reviews of this subject indicate that approximately 30 percent of patients return to work during the six months after discharge from a mental hospital; however, only approximately 15 percent are still employed by the one year follow-up point (56). Clearly, patients with severe mental disorders requiring hospitalization face obstacles in both finding and keeping jobs. Vocational rehabilitation programs have been designed for the full spectrum of psychiatric patients' needs, ranging from those who require a sheltered workshop setting indefinitely, those who can graduate from a transitional employment program into the competitive marketplace (57), to those who can resume their regular job after gaining a remission of their disorder.

For mental patients who are capable of assuming full-time, competitive employment, few will have jobs waiting for them. As a result, *job placement* becomes a crucial linchpin for those who are ready to meet the challenge of the world of work. How patients present themselves at job interviews is a critical determinant of whether or not they obtain work. Psychiatric patients may find it difficult to know how to respond to questions about their personal circumstances and recent past. Four studies, including two found in the 1978–1984 literature search described above, have demonstrated that psychiatric patients can benefit from training in interview skills (58–61).

Also important are knowing how to solicit job leads and having the motivation and persistence to sustain a long and frustrating job search (62). The Job Finding Club combines several successful techniques in a packaged program or module (63). Key elements of the module include 1) the use of an environment conducive to motivating patients in their job search, 2) use of reinforcement strategies, 3) a breakdown of the tasks involved in finding a job, and 4) the training of skills needed to find a job. To adapt this model to meet the needs of the psychiatrically disabled, it was necessary to increase the daily structure of the program, including daily goal-setting activities, and to develop remedial training in job-seeking skills. The Job Finding Club has been developed and evaluated at the West Los Angeles VA Medical Center (Brentwood Division) under a self-help and skill-building framework. Based on function rather than form, the services and activities of the program are directed by the maxim, "Does it get jobs?" There are three distinct segments in the Job Club—

training in job-seeking skills, the job search itself, and follow-up and job maintenance. While the program has no time limit, participants spend an average of 24 days in the program.

Training in job-seeking skills. During the first week of the program, patients participate in an intensive six-hour-per-day workshop designed to assess and train basic job-finding skills. The curriculum includes identifying sources of job leads, contacting job leads, filling out employment applications and resumes, participating in job interviews, and the use of public transportation. Instruction is competency based, with trainers using programmed materials, didactic instruction, role playing, and real life training exercises. Whenever possible, the program uses materials and situations that the client will face during the job search. For example, patients practice completing bona fide job applications and contacting actual sources for job leads. Patients' progress is continually monitored and additional instruction is provided to those who fall behind or present special training needs.

Job search. After completing the job-seeking skills workshop, patients begin the job search. The program provides work areas, secretarial support, and current job leads. These leads are gleaned from newspaper want ads, yellow pages, employment notices, civil service announcements, and weekly visits by state job placement counselors from two different agencies. Patients participate on a full-day basis. A daily intensive goal-setting session is conducted with each patient to plan job search activities. During this session counselors and patients identify the most advantageous options for the day's job search. They also develop outcome expectations for the daily activities, set a time line for accomplishment of the task, and carry out problem solving of potential stumbling blocks that may be encountered during the day. Patients are expected to keep a log of their daily job-seeking activities and account for their time in the program.

Another component of this phase involves teaching patients how to manage daily problems, including the stress of looking for employment. Supportive, goal-directed counseling is provided as needed. This may include assistance in finding housing and reliable transportation in the community, adjusting to work hours, and learning to interact with others. This phase lasts until the patient secures a job or leaves the program.

Follow-up and job-maintenance activities. Job Finding Club graduates may attend a weekly session that teaches methods to deal with problems that may threaten job security. Training adheres to a problem-solving model of specifying solutions to an identified issue and then role playing those solutions with feedback, before the client uses the approach in his work setting. Training issues are identified by the participants and may include learning how to get along with others on the job, managing psychiatric symptoms, and improving daily living situations. Graduates may also return to the program if they lose their jobs or wish to upgrade their positions.

Evaluation of the club. Fifty-seven percent of the 97 patients who participated in the program during the first eight months of operation secured employment, and another 10 percent entered full-time job training programs. Twelve percent of the patients voluntarily dropped out of the program during the first week of job-finding skills training, and an additional 10 percent of the patients dropped out after the first week when they were engaged in the actual job search. Eleven percent of the patients were returned to their wards by Job Finding Club staff because of reappearing symptoms that interfered with participation.

Participants spent an average of 23.9 working days in the program (range, 1–140 days). The average program stay for clients finding jobs was 12 days longer than for those who left the program employed.

The jobs secured fell into the following categories:

- 34 percent   clerical and sales positions
- 25 percent   service occupations
- 11 percent   professional
- 7 percent   machine trades
- 5.5 percent   benchwork jobs
- 5.5 percent   structural work jobs
- 12 percent   miscellaneous occupations

Job leads included the following:

- 39 percent   newspaper ads
- 22 percent   assistance from rehabilitation counselor
- 14 percent   help from a friend
- 10 percent   yellow pages
- 8 percent   civil service announcements
- 4 percent   private employment agencies
- 2 percent   unions
- 2 percent   walk-ins

There was no relationship between the type of job obtained and the source of the job lead (64).

Six-month follow-up data were collected on 74 percent of the 65 patients who entered jobs or job training from the program. The percentage of people employed 30, 60, 90, and 180 days after leaving the program was 80 percent, 75 percent, 80 percent, and 67.5 percent, respectively. Ten patients switched jobs during this time; and of these, six returned to the Job Finding Club for assistance. Of the patients who switched jobs, two were fired or laid off, five left their job for a better position, two found new work after symptom exacerbation forced them to leave their original positions, and one patient moved to a new location where he found work.

Of the 13 patients who were unemployed at the six-month follow-up, 4 lost their jobs because of psychiatric symptoms that interfered with their work, 4 quit their positions because of dissatisfaction with the job, 3 were fired, and 1 lost his job because of medical illness requiring hospitalization. Of the 25 patients who left the Job Finding Club without a successful placement, none of the individuals had found a job six months later.

Job outcomes have remained stable since the club's initiation. Out of a total referred patient group of approximately 300, 65 percent of the participants obtained jobs or entered vocational educational programs, and of this group, 65 percent were still employed at the six-month follow-up. Youth and absence of positive symptoms correlated with the ability to find jobs, as older patients and patients with positive symptoms were less likely to obtain a job. Previous work history and education did not predict the likelihood of finding employment, but did affect the type of jobs secured.

COMMON FEATURES AND ATTRIBUTES OF EFFECTIVE TREATMENT MODULES

The chronic mentally ill population needs medical and psychiatric treatment, housing, vocational rehabilitation, recreational programs, financial assistance, social rehabilitation, and crisis intervention services. As a result of deinstitutionalization, communities are now responsible for providing for the care and treatment of a large percentage of the severely mentally ill. Until recently, local community mental health programs were ill prepared to meet their responsibilities for the long-term treatment and needs of the chronically mentally ill.

Resource Book for Psychiatric Rehabilitation

NIMH initiated the Community Support Program (CSP) in 1977 to upgrade treatment and rehabilitation for deinstitutionalized and new young chronic psychiatric patients. This program's goal was to stimulate and assist states and communities in the development of community based services for the long term mentally ill. As part of the NIMH efforts, the Rehabilitation, Research, and Training Center in Mental Illness developed the *Resource Book for Psychiatric Rehabilitation: Elements of Service for the Mentally Ill* (65). The aim of the book was to help model community support programs, nominated from throughout the country, to operationalize their treatment and rehabilitation activities into modular form. Highly specified and replicable descriptions of program elements are provided in the *Resource Book* for approximately 50 CSP model programs across the nation. Elements were classified by the spectrum of services recommended by the NIMH CSP, including psychosocial services; outreach activities; entitlement assistance; 24-hour crisis intervention; community involvement in community support system planning; continuous support services; advocacy; case management; back-up support for families, friends, and the community; and medical and mental health care. Each service area comprised multiple treatment components; for example, under psychosocial services would be listed social skills training and vocational and prevocational rehabilitation. Hence, the *Resource Book* catalogued exemplary elements of service according to the component that best represented its primary functional purpose. Each component category of the *Resource Book* contained multiple elements; for example, sheltered workshops, job club, and transitional employment programs were elements of the vocational and prevocational rehabilitation component.

The information included for each exemplary program element in the *Resource Book* was obtained through an interactive process. Nominations of exemplary programs were received from a variety of sources, including each state's Community Support Program director, mental health professionals, consumers, researchers, and a computerized search of the literature. In organizing the format and style for the *Resource Book*, the authors wrote a few sample entries describing the characteristics of exemplary program elements and sent them for review to a national sample of the potential users of the book. Feedback was obtained on what additional information should be included as well as on the information that was redundant or nonessential for practitioners' use in implementing elements in their settings. This feedback was incorporated into the design of the questionnaires that were sent out to the nominated programs.

Information was solicited from program staff via the questionnaire on their service element's effectiveness, procedures, administrative structure, staffing, budget, client characteristics, and community characteristics. Programs were also asked to send any additional information along with the questionnaire that might be useful to the authors in writing a richly descriptive entry for the *Resource Book* (for example, annual reports, advisory board meeting minutes). When this information was received, the questionnaires were screened for completeness and the elements for documented effectiveness. Many programs received follow-up calls from the authors to obtain more specific information on the program element itself. After the operationalization of each entry into modular form was completed, the draft was sent back to the program for approval. The final approved and revised drafts were then sent to the Advisory Panel for the *Resource Book*. The Advisory Panel consisted of mental health service providers, mental health administrators, consumers, and researchers, and they screened and approved entries for their potential utility and exportability.

The *Resource Book* was designed for practitioners, administrators, and policymakers who work with the chronic mentally ill. Program elements were grouped and cross-indexed by their principal focus, and an annotated bibliography of articles and books useful in the implementation of model programs was provided. In addition, a checklist of steps to follow when implementing an entry is included in the book. A questionnaire asking users to evaluate elements in the *Resource Book* that they tried to implement is sent out to gather data that will enable the authors to revise the book to better meet users' needs. Thus, each subsequent edition of the *Resource Book* will reflect the accumulated experience and empirical value stemming from practitioners attempting to replicate exemplary elements of service for the chronic mentally ill.

Structure of Model Programs

Leona Bachrach (25) identified eight common features of effective programs for chronic mental patients:

1. Chronic patients are the target group—priority is assigned to the most severely impaired.
2. Linkage with other resources—in addition to case management, patients receive additional special services (for example, residential services, vocational rehabilitation, and so forth).
3. Functional integrity—programs providing a full range of functions— at least equivalent to the range of services available in institutions.
4. Individually tailored treatment—this includes case management and 24-hour crisis intervention.
5. Cultural relevance and specificity—programs conform to local realities of the communities.

6. Specially trained staff.
7. Hospital liaison.
8. Internal evaluation.

The authors of the *Resource Book* reviewed the entries of service elements drawn from the national sample of model programs to identify attributes common to these programs. Many of the features identified by Leona Bachrach were applicable to the programs in the *Resource Book*. Effective programs typically were private nonprofit corporations devoted solely to the care of the chronic mentally ill. Successful programs were directed by a variety of professionals (for example, psychiatrists, psychologists), administrators (for example, MBAs), registered nurses, occupational therapists, and social workers who had career commitments to the chronic mentally ill. Many of these programs were located near universities and made extensive use of undergraduate and graduate students as volunteers, which permitted a wider range of individually tailored services at low cost. Interagency agreements were frequently established (for example, with the police department, mental health clinics, hospitals, and local business) to insure smooth delivery of comprehensive services to the patients. Programs provided multiple service elements, typically with a case manager linking the client with appropriate services.

Program effectiveness was evaluated at least annually by the programs nominated for the *Resource Book*. Measures included rehospitalization rates, exacerbation of symptoms, goal attainment, employment, and independent living outcomes. Measures of success included patients' stability as well as progress to higher levels of functioning (for example, a patient who remained in a supervised apartment would be considered a success, as would a patient who "graduated" to a satellite apartment).

Delivery of Services in Model Programs

Services within the model elements in the *Resource Book* were typically tailored to the needs of the individual. Upon admission to the program, a functional assessment was conducted identifying the patient's strengths and weaknesses. Treatment goals were determined from this assessment, with input from the patient. For most patients enrolled in exemplary programs, three to four short-term goals were worked on concurrently.

Services followed a standard curriculum format with scheduled activities and responsibilities. Day treatment programs and social and independent living skills training programs often utilized a manual in which skills were taught in a sequential manner. Psychosocial clubs, vocational programs, and residential programs in the *Resource Book* had scheduled activities and responsibilities. Staff members received training and attended in-service training on a regular basis. Initial training of new employees often included instruction on first aid, psychotropic medications, and crisis intervention techniques.

Leona Bachrach (25) identified the need for strategies that could translate model-derived knowledge into systems-related actions. The interactive process utilized by the authors of the *Resource Book* to obtain specific information on program elements or modules provides one such strategy. It is hoped that these modules can be readily incorporated into existing programs and modified to meet the particular needs, resources, and constraints of local agencies and facilities (65).

POLICY IMPLICATIONS

If our premise has merit, that innovations in the delivery of services to chronic mental patients are facilitated by the design of treatment modules, then what can be done by administrators, legislators, and other policymakers in the mental health and human service systems? One starting point would be to establish research development and utilization units within the mental health system. Such a unit would have the following purposes and functions:

1. To cull new procedures and elements that have been found particularly effective from the literature and conferences and from ongoing communication and interaction with innovators throughout a region, state, and country.
2. To design and develop new procedures and techniques in league with clinicians and service settings located in nearby or adjacent hospitals, clinics, and mental health centers. There are many missed opportunities to develop and disseminate innovative packages or modules from the creative and effective work carried out in obscurity by dedicated and experienced line-level clinicians.
3. To adapt and fashion modules for distinct treatment and rehabilitation goals, populations, and settings, perhaps on the basis of a contract made with an agency, institution, or program that has the need for such a module. These modules may be fabricated from existing methods or abstracted from much wider and more comprehensive programs. The challenges in fabricating modules are a) to simplify and operationalize them so they are easily learned and adopted by clinicians and b) to ensure that they fit well into existing comprehensive programs.

4. To assist clinicians in adopting innovations, from new pharmaco-therapy strategies to psychosocial modules. This function can be carried out through linkages with in-service training faculty, provision of workshops, and on-the-job training. Examples of effective and creative educational methods and the obstacles and resistance to innovation that must be overcome have been described elsewhere (24, 66).
5. To evaluate the impact of innovations that are being implemented by actively soliciting feedback from clinicians, whose use of those innovative methods can guide further refinements and changes in the methods themselves. Thus, an interactional process can be set up between the research development and utilization unit and its clinician "consumers" such that constant tailoring and evolution of modules and other innovations take place. This is the aim of the *Resource Book* described above.
6. To strive to establish model or demonstration units in which organizational structure, roles, and operating principles have effectively supported innovative and comprehensive residential and community programs. Such demonstration programs could form the infrastructure for testing the value of new service elements or modules in upgrading overall comprehensive programs. Model units within regional or state systems could minimize training and start-up costs for adoptees by establishing an integrated program based on the best research and consultation concerning presently available technologies.

Research utilization in mental health can take cues from successful experiences in technology transfer found in other areas of our society. For example, in agriculture, field agents of a state's university extension services work hand-in-hand with farmers to help them adopt new seeds, fertilizers, pesticides, equipment, and planting and harvesting techniques. Another example comes from the pharmaceutical industry, where "detail" salespersons visit physicians in their offices and hospitals to provide educational information on new drugs and facilitate adoption of them.

If we take seriously the concept of a research utilization specialist for fostering change and innovation in mental health practices, then what are some of this persons's characteristics? The research utilization specialist would have to come from clinician's ranks, yet possess research know-how and sophistication. The specialist would have to be able to discriminate statistical significance from social and clinical significance in sifting through research publications of new methods. Communication and relationship skills would have to be high in the specialist's repertoire, and this person would have to be able to demonstrate his or her competence to practitioners in the "trenches" by modeling the very techniques being disseminated with clients and patients. The specialist would have to possess a keen appreciation of active learning and teaching techniques and not hope to introduce new methods through dry and clinically removed classroom training. Thus, clinical skills would have to be kept sharply honed, as well as negotiation skills for establishing contracts or agreements with agencies and programs wanting services from the research development and utilization unit.

To establish a niche in the existing mental health service network, an innovative program or module, like any other commodity, needs to be marketed and sold. Although the concept of selling a product may be new to human service providers, it has already taken hold in the marketing of hospital and clinic services in the private sector. Newspaper, television, and radio advertisements regularly evoke interest among people wanting to quit smoking or drinking, get their teeth fixed, or have a baby. There is no reason why innovations in mental health cannot be similarly marketed, and done so on the basis of their empirical validation. After all, if aspirin can be sold by expounding technical data on its buffering action in the stomach, why can't a new psychosocial treatment module be sold by virtue of its documented effectiveness in reducing relapse rates and improving quality of life? The research utilization specialist, then, will need to have or to obtain marketing skills as well.

The cadre of research utilization specialists would also have to be able to set goals realistically and incrementally in the context of well-defined time frames. In facilitating the change process, specialists would have to maintain flexibility, cope with institutional constraints, deal with sources of conflict, and maintain support from the host agency's power structure.

In shaping a shared vision with administrators and clinical leaders desiring to introduce innovation, the research utilization specialist should convince policymakers and program directors to buy into the change process by actively participating in it. This could be done by obtaining a pledge from such busy organization leaders to spend "an hour a day to keep stagnation at bay." Even an hour a week of a leader's making rounds and encouraging those line-level staff who are involved in innovative efforts can powerfully reinforce the change process. It is also important for change agents to form close partnerships with local agency "champions" for innovation. Such champions can be found in every agency, although their capabilities for serving as facilitators and spokespersons for adopting new methods may be latent or dormant. Championing new methods should come from employees who are perceived as outstanding clinicians by their peers and who have high informal status within the organization. Sociometric methods could be used to select them, and both formal and social rewards could sustain their involvement.

No matter how skilled and persuasive the research utilization specialist might be, there are factors within the organization that need to be stimulated to promote desired change. For example, special incentives need to be offered to clinicians and programs that are willing to "go the extra mile" in adopting an innovation. At Camarillo State Hospital in California, the management team offered an extra budget allotment to any ward that implemented a demonstrably effective token economy or credit system for its patients. This not only promoted the adoption of a new technique, but also helped to insure that the methods would not be introduced in "token" fashion because of insufficient funds to purchase backup reinforcers for the patients. In a time of severely limited budgets, this budget supplement not only supported an innovation directly, but also provided tangible and symbolic reinforcement to those staff who organized and delivered consistent programming.

Stories of the failure of initially successful and effective innovative programs abound; thus, the staff of the research development and utilization unit must attend to the maintenance as well as the introduction of innovations. Failure sometimes comes when key clinicians or program leaders depart from an agency. Other reasons for failure come from the splits or conflicts that develop between the values and goals of the innovative program's staff and those of their parent agency. For example, some highly successful programs for rehabilitating severely impaired developmentally disabled clients have run aground when the more academically oriented program leadership wanted to continue to experiment and refine program elements, while the board of directors (who were mostly parents of the clients) were content with the status quo (67).

Another example of failure of an innovation to take root was an effort to introduce parent education groups for low-income families designated as high risk for abuse, neglect, developmental delay, or emotional disturbance. Funding was easily secured and enthusiasm was voiced by community professionals concerned with the psychologic health of families. However, the expected torrent of referrals never materialized, and it became apparent that there were implicit discrepancies between the professional's and client's perceptions of needs (68). Similar innovative parent training programs foundered because they ran afoul of competing values of client recruitment with other agencies within the human service system (69, 70).

It is imperative the research development and utilization unit take pains to establish and maintain a consistent frame of reference and a common pursuit of goals with the leadership of those agencies that interact with the program targeted for innovation. This is as important as the working relationship with practitioners undertaking the innovation. As has been pointed out by organizational sociologists:

> A mental health service delivery system is conceptualized as a set of mental health-related service units that interact with one another at a given moment in time within a bounded geographic area. An essential feature of these systems is that they consist of a number of stakeholder groups that have different power positions and different vested interests in the local community. These groups include local government, state officials and their organizations, hospitals, private for-profit and not-for-profit agencies, self-help organizations, families and clients. Each of these groups are involved in a struggle for limited resources. At a given moment in time, a dominant coalition of powerful groups exists. The dominant coalition consists of those groups or organizations whose interests are considered in defining the system's goals. Each group or organization attempts to impose its preferences on the system. Local systems operate within constraints established by the state and federal government and by economic factors such as insurance reimbursement contingencies. (71)

The rivalry and conflicts in values and goals between supposedly cooperative service agencies are highlighted by the state's vocational rehabilitation programs and mental health delivery systems. Instead of pooling resources and expertise, their differing mandates often create barriers to collaboration. The vocational rehabilitation programs are justified and funded on the basis of rehabilitation outcomes judged successful if clients are placed relatively quickly in competitive jobs. In contrast, mental health programs are funded and justified on the basis of serving the full range of long-term needs of psychiatrically impaired patients with social and occupational deficits. Many psychiatric patients are very hard to place in jobs, because of their symptoms, bizarre behavior, social inadequacies, and vulnerability to relapse. Vocational rehabilitation counselors are reluctant to accept referrals from mental health programs if those people are likely to remain on their case load for a prolonged period and if they have a small chance of responding to traditional counseling procedures. If research utilization specialists are aware of these interagency conflicts in mission, they can more easily promote an innovation such as the Job Finding Club, which incorporates a set of techniques to facilitate the placement of mentally ill clients.

Maintaining innovative programs, and keeping them vital and effective, forces the research utilization specialist to summon a wide variety of skills in addition to personal endurance. Key among these are shaping and sustaining the performance of staff over the long haul and linking staff behavior to empirical feedback loops of on-going program evaluation.

The social and clinical value of innovative elements and modules ultimately depends not only on technologic efficacy, but also on the ability of the utilization specialist to cope with the sociopolitics of institutional change and resistance.

As we ponder our next steps in bringing effective new treatment and rehabilitation techniques to our patients, let us be sustained by the words of this anonymous philosopher:

> It is not the critic who counts, not the man who points how the strong man stumbles, or where the doer of deeds could have done them better. The credit belongs to the man or woman who is actually in the arena, whose face is marred by dust and sweat and blood, who strives violently, who errs and comes short again and again, who knows the great enthusiasms, the great devotion and spends himself or herself in a worthy cause, who at the best knows in the end the triumph of high achievement, and who at the worst if he or she fails, at least fails while daring greatly so that his or her place shall never be with those cold and timid souls who know neither victory nor defeat.

REFERENCES

1. Paul GL, Lentz RJ: Psychosocial Treatment of the Chronic Mental Patient. Cambridge, MA, Harvard University Press, 1977
2. Liberman RP, Foy DW: Psychiatric rehabilitation for chronic mental patients. Psychiatric Annals 13:539–545, 1983
3. Leff JP, Hirsch SR, Gaind R, et al: Life events and maintenance therapy in schizophrenic relapse. Br J Psychiatry 123:659–668, 1973
4. Vaughn CE, Snyder KS, Freeman W, et al: Family factors in schizophrenic relapse: a replication. Schizophr Bull 8:425–426, 1982
5. Leff JP, Vaughn CE: The role of maintenance therapy and relatives' expressed emotion in relapse of schizophrenia: a two year follow-up. Br J Psychiatry 139:102–104, 1981
6. Hogarty GE, Schooler NR, Ulrich R, et al: Fluphenazine and social therapy in the aftercare of schizophrenic patients. Arch Gen Psychiatry 36:1283–1295, 1979
7. Liberman RP, Wallace CJ, Vaughn CE, et al: Social and family factors in the course of schizophrenia: toward an interpersonal problem-solving therapy for schizophrenics and their relatives, in Psychotherapy of Schizophrenia: Current Status and New Directions. Edited by Strauss J, Fleck S, Bowers M. New York, Plenum Press, 1980
8. Nuechterlein KH, Dawson ME: Information processing and attentional functioning in the developmental cause of schizophrenic disorders. Schizophr Bull 10:160–202, 1984

9. Barter J: Successful community programming for the chronic mental patient, in The Chronic Mental Patient: Problems, Solutions, and Recommendations for a Public Policy. Edited by Talbott J. Washington, DC, American Psychiatric Association, 1978

10. Diamond RJ: Increasing medication compliance in young adult chronic psychiatric patients, in Advances in Treating the Young Adult Chronic Patient. Edited by Pepper B, Ryglewicz H. New Directions for Mental Health Services, no. 21. San Francisco, Jossey-Bass, 1984

11. Wallace CJ, Boone SE, Donahoe CP, et al: The chronically mentally disabled: social and independent living skills training, in Behavioral Treatment of Adult Disorders. Edited by Barlow D. New York, Guilford Press, 1984

12. Marder S, Mintz J, Van Putten T, et al: The effects of low dose fluphenazine on relapse and side effects in chronic outpatient schizophrenics. Paper presented at the Annual Meeting of the American Psychiatric Association, Los Angeles, CA, May 1984

13. Kane JM, Woerner M, Weinhold P, et al: A prospective study of tardive dyskinesia development: preliminary results. J Clin Psychopharmacol 2:345–349, 1982

14. Kane JM, Rifkin A, Woerner M, et al: Low dose neuroleptic treatment of outpatient schizophrenics. I. Preliminary results for relapse rates. Arch Gen Psychiatry 40:893–896, 1983

15. Carpenter WT, Stephens JH, Rey AC, et al: Early intervention vs. continuous pharmacotherapy of schizophrenia. Psychopharmacol Bull 18:21–23, 1982

16. Herz MI, Szymanski HV, Simon JC: Intermittent medication for stable schizophrenic outpatients: an alternative to maintenance medication. Am J Psychiatry 139:918–922, 1982

17. Test MA, Stein LI: Training in community living, in Alternatives to Mental Hospital Treatment. Edited by Stein LI, Test MA. New York, Plenum Press, 1978

18. Glasscote RM, Cumming E, Rutman ED, et al: Rehabilitating the Mentally Ill in the Community: A Study of Psychosocial Rehabilitation Centers. Washington, DC, American Psychiatric Association, 1971

19. Stein LI, Test MA: Alternatives to mental hospital treatment. Arch Gen Psychiatry 37:392–397, 1980

20. Beard JH, Malamud TJ, Rossman E: Psychiatric rehabilitation and long term rehospitalization rates: the findings of two research studies. Schizophr Bull 4:622–635, 1978

21. Matthews SM, Roper MT, Mosher LR, et al: A non-neuroleptic treatment for schizophrenia: analysis of the two year post discharge risk of relapse. Schizophr Bull 7:221–256, 1981

22. Fairweather GW, Sanders DJ, Maynerd H, et al: Community Life for the Mentally Ill. New York, Aldine Press, 1969
23. Meyerson AT: What are the barriers or obstacles to treatment and care of the chronically disabled mentally ill?, in The Chronic Mental Patient: Problems, Solutions, and Recommendations for a Public Policy. Edited by Talbott JA. Washington, DC, American Psychiatric Association, 1978
24. Liberman RP: Sociopolitics of behavioral programs in institutions and community agencies. Analysis and Intervention in Developmental Disabilities 3:131–159, 1983
25. Bachrach LL: Overview: model programs for chronic mental patients. Am J Psychiatry 137:1023–1031, 1980
26. Paul GL: The impact of public policy and decision making on the development and dissemination of science-based practices in mental institutions: playing poker with everything wild, in Psychological Research, Public Policy and Practice: Towards a Productive Partnership. Edited by Kasschau RA, Rehm L, Ullman LP. New York, Praeger, 1985
27. Wallace CJ, Boone SE, Donahoe CP, et al: The chronically mentally disabled: social and independent living skills training, in Behavioral Treatment of Adult Disorders. Edited by Barlow D. New York, Guilford Press, 1984
28. Liberman RP, Falloon IRH, Wallace CJ: Drug-psychosocial interactions in the treatment of schizophrenia, in The Chronically Mentally Ill: Research and Services. Edited by Mirabi M. New York, SP Medical and Scientific Books, 1984
29. Liberman RP: Social factors in schizophrenia, in Psychiatry Update—1982. Edited by Grinspoon L. Washington, DC, American Psychiatric Press, 1982
30. Hirschfeld RMA, Klerman GL, Clayton PJ, et al: Assessing personality: effects of the depressive state on trait measurement. Am J Psychiatry 140:695–699, 1983
31. Presly AS, Grubb AB, Semple D: Predictors of successful rehabilitation in long-stay patients. Acta Psychiatr Scand 66:83–88, 1982
32. Sylph JA, Ross HE, Kedward HB: Social disabiity in chronic psychiatric patients. Am J Psychiatry 134:1391–1394, 1978
33. Linn MW, Klett J, Caffey FM: Foster home characteristics and psychiatric patient outcome. Arch Gen Psychiatry 37:129–132, 1980
34. Vaughn CE, Snyder KS, Freeman W, et al: Family factors in schizophrenic relapse. Arch Gen Psychiatry 41:1169–1177, 1984
35. Monti PM, Curran JP, Corriveau DP, et al: Effects of social skills training groups with psychiatric patients. J Consult Clin Psychol 48:241–248, 1980

36. Monti PM, Fink E, Norman W, et al: Effects of social skills training groups and social skills bibliotherapy with psychiatric patients. J Consult Clin Psychol 47:189–191, 1979
37. Kelly JA, Urey JR, Patterson JT: Improving heterosocial conversational skills of male psychiatric patients through a small group training procedure. Behav Res Ther 11:179–193, 1980
38. Nelson GL, Cone JD: Multiple baseline analysis of a token economy for psychiatric inpatients. J Appl Behav Anal 12:255–271, 1979
39. Liberman RP, King LW, DeRisi WJ, et al: Personal Effectiveness: Guiding People to Assert Themselves and Improve Their Social Skills. Champaign, IL, Research Press, 1975
40. Foy DW, Wallace CJ, Liberman RP: Advances in social skills training for chronic mental patients, in Advances in Clinical Behavior Therapy. Edited by Craig KD, McMahon RJ. New York, Brunner/Mazel, 1983
41. Massel HK, Bowen L, Mosk MD, et al: A comparison of procedures for training conversational skills in chronic schizophrenics. Paper presented at the Association for the Advancement of Behavior Therapy, Philadelphia, PA, November 1984
42. Liberman RP, King LW, DeRisi WJ: Behavior analysis and therapy in community mental health, in Handbook of Behavior Therapy and Modification. Edited by Leitenburg H. Englewood Cliffs, NJ, Prentice Hall, 1976
43. Liberman RP, Kuehnel T, Kuehnel J, et al: The BAM Project: from conception to dissemination, in Community Health: A Behavioral-Ecological Perspective. Edited by Slotnick RS, Jeger AM. New York, Plenum Press, 1982
44. Falloon IRH, Liberman RP: Behavioral family interventions in the management of chronic schizophrenia, in Family Therapy in Schizophrenia. Edited by McFarlane WR. New York, Guilford Press, 1983
45. Creer T: Schizophrenia at Home. London, National Schizophrenic Fellowship, 1974
46. Brown G, Birley JLP, Wing JK: Influence of family life on the course of schizophrenia. Br J Psychiatry 121:241–258, 1972
47. Snyder KS, Liberman RP: Family assessment and intervention with schizophrenics at risk for relapse, in New Developments in Interventions with Families of Schizophrenics. Edited by Goldstein MJ. New Directions for Mental Health Services, no. 12 San Francisco, Jossey-Bass, 1981
48. Falloon IRH, McGill C, Boyd J: Behavioral Family Management. Baltimore, Johns Hopkins University Press, 1984
49. Falloon, IRH, Boyd JL, McGill CW, et al: Family management in the

prevention of exacerbations of schizophrenia: a controlled study. N Engl J Med 306:1437–1440, 1982

50. Brenner MH: Mental Illness and the Economy. Cambridge, MA, Harvard University Press, 1973
51. Hagen DQ: The relationship between job loss and physical and mental illness. Hosp Community Psychiatry 34:438–441, 1983
52. Greco MA, Stein LI: An alternative to hospitalization programming: the contribution of a rehabilitation approach. Rehabiliation Counseling Bulletin 24:85–93, 1980
53. Lehman AF, Ward NC, Linn LS: Chronic mental patients: the quality of life issue. Am J Psychiatry 133:796–823, 1983
54. Goldstrom I, Manderscheid R: The chronically mentally ill: a descriptive analysis from the uniform client data instrument. Community Support Services Journal 2:4–9, 1982
55. Strauss JS, Hafez H: Clinical questions and "real" research. Am J Psychiatry 138:1592–1597, 1981
56. Anthony WA, Cohen MR, Vitalo R: The measurement of rehabilitation outcome. Schizophr Bull 4:365–383, 1978
57. Beard JH: Industry and the vocational rehabilitation of the disabled mental patient. Paper presented at the Annual Meeting of the President's Committee on Employment of the Handicapped, Washington, DC, April 1982
58. Kiel EC, Barbee JR: Training the disadvantaged job interviewee. Vocational Guidance Quarterly 22:50–56, 1973
59. Vernardos MG, Harris MB: Job interview training with rehabilitation clients. J Appl Psychol 58:365–367, 1973
60. Furman W, Geller M, Simon SJ, et al: The use of a behavioral rehearsal procedure for teaching job interview skills to psychiatric patients. Behav Res Ther 10:157–167, 1979
61. Kelly JA, Laughlin C, Claiborne M, et al: A group procedure for teaching job interview skills to formerly hospitalized psychiatric patients. Behav Res Ther 10:299–310, 1979
62. Watts FN: Employment in Theory and Practice of Psychiatric Rehabilitation. Edited by Watts FN, Bennett DH. New York, Wiley, 1983
63. Azrin NH, Besalel VA: Job Club Counselors Manual: A Behavioral Approach to Vocational Counseling. Baltimore, University Park Press, 1980
64. Jacobs HE, Kardashian S, Kreinbring RK, et al: A skills oriented model for facilitating employment among psychiatrically disabled persons. Rehabilitation Counseling Bulletin 28:87–96, 1984
65. Liberman RP, Kuehnel TG, Phipps CC, et al: Resource Book for Psy-

chiatric Rehabilitation: Elements of Services for the Mentally Ill. Los Angeles, University of California Press, 1985

66. Liberman RP: Social and political challenges to the development of behavioral programs in organizations, in Trends in Behavior Therapy. Edited by Sjoden PO, Dockens WS, Bates S. New York, Academic Press, 1979

67. Graziano AM: Clinical innovation and the mental health power structure: A social case history. Am Psychol 24:10–18, 1969

68. Rosenberg MS, Repucci ND, Linney JA: Issues in the implementation of human service programs: examples from a parent training project for high risk families. Analysis and Intervention in Developmental Disabilities 3:215–226, 1983

69. Ball T, Jarvis RM, Pease SSF: Interinstitutional misadventure in a training program for parents of retarded children: who gets caught in the middle? Analysis and Interventions in Developmental Disabilities 3:239–248, 1983

70. Barber K, Barber M, Clark HB: Establishing a community-oriented group home and ensuring its survival: a case study of failure. Analysis and Intervention in Developmental Disabilities 3:227–238, 1983

71. Grosky D: Assessing the Effects of Local Mental Health Delivery Systems (Grant no. R-01-MH 38 887). Rockville, MD, National Institute of Mental Health, 1985

CHAPTER 6

Chronic Mental Illness:
A Problem in Politics

JOSEPH J. BEVILACQUA, PH.D.
JOHN H. NOBLE, JR., PH.D.

In this chapter we purposefully and consciously associate chronic mental illness with politics. Professionals are usually uncomfortable in identifying themselves with politics, except when it involves guild interest—the rights, prerogatives, and financing of professional practice. Thus, it is easier for professionals to advocate for client interests when both guild and client interests are intertwined. Because this is so, the chronic mentally ill receive little positive attention. Without means to pay for professional services themselves, they have to rely on underfinanced public programs for clinical treatment and supportive services.

Until the relationship between chronic mental illness and the political process is faced squarely, we will not be able to move toward implementation of meaningful programs nor be able to resolve in a satisfactory manner *the* major mental health problem in this country. Politics and the political process intervene in the economy to circumvent market forces in order to assure the financing of specific communal objectives that would not otherwise be met (1). Since there is no natural market for serving the chronic mentally ill in the United States, or in any other country for that matter, government and the political process are the only way to address their needs.

We are grateful to Donald K. Jones, M.D., and Karen Mallem, M.B.A., for their assistance in preparing this chapter.

But declaring this to be the fact does not make it happen. The professions, the universities which train the professions, and the constituencies of chronic mentally ill persons themselves and their families must act in concert if meaningful programs of treatment and care are to be created and sustained or a beginning made in resolving the problem of chronic mental illness in the United States. How this is done is what politics is all about. The reference to politics is in no way pejorative. It simply reflects how interest group democracy operates.

This paper addresses four questions:

- What are the obstacles to implementing programs for the chronic mentally ill?
- What are the financial and control issues relating to services for the chronic mentally ill?
- What are the legal issues associated with providing services for the chronic mentally ill?
- What are the problems created by societal stereotyping of persons with chronic mental illness?

It is necessary to take a political perspective to obtain answers to these questions, because they all involve issues of power, status, and public resources. Chronic mental illness, although not associated exclusively with any particular social class, becomes the responsibility of the public sector because chronic mentally ill persons, if not already poor, eventually fall into poverty. In addition, treatment of the chronic mentally ill requires a broad-based, multiorganizational infrastructure that is beyond the capacity of the private sector to build and sustain.

Chronic mental illness presents a host of needs that transcend the usual array of agency- and discipline-specific solutions. Sustaining chronic mentally ill persons in the least-restrictive environment appropriate to their needs requires many inputs—clinical services, including medication; income support; housing; psychosocial rehabilitation; and case management and advocacy. The challenge is not technical knowledge. Our knowledge about how to treat and care for the chronic mentally ill is sufficient. We know what works from any number of studies (2). The challenge is political acumen—how to move ahead in the face of obstacles to acquisition of the necessary resources and to successful implementation of programs.

The first step is to recognize the obstacles. By doing so, we become more capable of implementing the approaches that work, using the tools required to make them work. In this view, politics involves government as well as professional and constituency group activities—all directed toward the deployment of the necessary technical and monetary resources to implement approaches that work. When this is recognized, it forces us to look outside our usual sphere of responsibility and control to stimulate actions to obtain all the necessary technical and monetary resources needed to do the job.

THE OBSTACLES

Current Professional Education and Practice

The political forces that create change cut across many sectors. Let us briefly look at professional training within the traditional mental health disciplines of medicine, nursing, psychology, and social work and question how we educate and prepare ourselves for practice. Take, for example, the discipline of social work. According to a report by Rubin (3) for the Council on Social Work Education, 80 percent of graduate students aspire to the private practice of psychotherapy within five years of graduation. Private practice is where there is money, prestige, and the freedom to be selective in the choice of clients. Surely the increasing number of faculty members who maintain a private psychotherapy practice on the side must influence the role modeling of students.

This development in a discipline that has traditionally focused on the psychosocial and environmental components of illness and social problems reflects both economic forces and government inaction. Money considerations and the laissez-faire of government funding have encouraged social work to provide training in a form of practice that cannot respond to the service needs of chronic mentally ill persons.

Just as social work has emulated the office-based, private practice of medicine as its preferred model, so nursing and psychology appear to be moving along a similar track. As a result, the very disciplines that are needed to successfully treat and care for the chronic mentally ill are removing themselves from the effort. They are disaffiliating themselves from the organizations and programs that create the infrastructure for serving the chronic mentally ill in community settings.

Just as devastating is the paucity of attention paid to chronic mental illness in the curricula of the mental health disciplines. How many professional schools that prepare mental health practitioners pay special attention to the service needs and the technology for serving the chronic mentally ill? Not many.

Two conclusions can be reached. First, the practice model being used in professional education is not conducive to organizing and drawing together the necessary technologies for dealing with chronic mental illness. The solo practice model, and perhaps worse, the current "corporatization" of practice in mental health, drive professionals away from contact with the chronic mentally ill. Second, the lack of focused attention on chronic mental illness in curriculum development within professional schools gives no foundation on which to build the necessary course content and research. Students do not learn about the appropriate technologies, nor do they obtain practice in their use.

Changing our pedagogic and practice structures will ultimately require political decisions. Such change is controlled by the interaction of government policies and the professional disciplines and their guilds. We know from the sociology of professions that when certain tasks lose favor within a particular profession, somebody else comes along to take over the "undesirable" work. Will this be the fate of the contemporary mental health disciplines with regard to the chronic mentally ill? Will a new profession or professions arise from necessity to serve the chronic mentally ill? The answer is contingent on both government action and the response of the professional disciplines and their guilds.

The obstacles to implementing programs for the chronic mentally ill that originate in the disciplines and their guilds are structural in nature. Removing them will require the kind of leveraging for change that comes only from political activity. With federal funds for professional education in mental health diminishing, the states are emerging as an important alternative source of funding. An important first step will have been taken if state government begins to ask how the state-funded universities are addressing such problems as chronic mental illness and if the legislative branch can be persuaded to appropriate funds to bring attention to these problems. The disciplines and their guilds will have to take the second step. If the mental health disciplines show no interest, there will be some new profession sure to emerge to fill the gap.

Government

When examining the activities of the different levels of government— federal, state, and local—we realize that, in the main, the chronic mentally ill have not received full attention from any of these levels. Since the founding of the National Institute of Mental Health (NIMH), the focus has rarely been on the chronic mentally ill. The exception occurred during the Carter Administration, when the community support program and the Mental Health Systems Act addressed some of the needs of this population. A national plan for the chronic mentally ill was completed by the U.S. Department of Health and Human Services (4) but never implemented. Generally, however, the federal government has not exhibited significant leadership with respect to funding of services for the chronic mentally ill. As a matter of fact, the U.S. Congress has excluded the adult psychiatric population, ages 22–64, from federal support while undergoing treatment in a free-standing psychiatric facility. Most of these patients are cared for in state mental hospitals, and the federal government did not wish to assure responsibility for financing their care as it did for the mentally retarded through Title XIX of the Social Security Act. This fact says much about the weakness of mental health constituencies at the federal level.

Leadership at the federal level has not been able to generate the kind of clout needed to gain financial support for the chronic mentally ill that it has for some other disabilities. This is because state government has traditionally paid for the basic care of chronic mentally ill persons, and the federal government recognized the opportunity to contain costs by avoiding, wherever possible, coverage of state institutional populations, largely prisoners and the chronic mentally ill. Unlike many other constituencies—most especially children—the elderly mentally ill have lacked the power to lay claim on federal resources. Thus, state general funds have been the primary source of funding for the adult psychiatric population, including the chronic mentally ill.

Lynn (5) succinctly describes the value system that largely explains why state services to the chronic mentally ill have been so problematic and in flux:

> Elected state officials have on the whole a greater sense of responsibility toward economy and efficiency in governmental operations than they do toward the effectiveness of coverage of human services. A composite view is "human services have no constituency. Their clients do not vote, at least not in large enough numbers to make a difference to the average legislator. The average voter is concerned about his or her taxes and wants assurances that revenues are not wasted." Even governors who have reputations as being "for" human services, such as Askew and Evans, could not ignore the economy issue, nor could the heads of their human service organizations.
>
> In short, fiscal discipline must be a primary objective of governors and legislators. They are continuously vulnerable to the charge that government operations are wasteful and insufficient. The passage of Proposition 13 in California and other tax eliminating legislation elsewhere only accentuates what have been generally true: Economy and efficiency are salient issues in the states and nothing is likely to alter that picture. (p 18)

To the extent that state government has seen opportunities to balance its budget by minimizing the cost of care to the psychiatrically impaired poor, that is, the chronic mentally ill, the states as well as the federal government have been able to secure cost savings and thus apparent economies and efficiencies in governmental operations. The general population of voters does not care, and the chronic mentally ill and their families do not have enough votes to make a difference!

As an offset to this political reality, the pattern of state mental health operations across the states is not encouraging. The "shelf life" of mental health commissioners is short. Each year one-third of the commissioners leave their jobs. This means that there is no sustained professional leadership. There is too little time to educate the governor and members of the legislature. In short, the term of the commissioner becomes one of crisis management. Too often time and energy are spent fighting scandals and media exposés bred of inadequate funding of programs. Thus, a vacuum comes to exist between the commissioner and the sources of constituency support that are needed to successfully administer the mental health agency. What is more, opportunities to improve the system and to make a persuasive case for better policies and budgets get lost amidst political infighting that does nothing to serve the legitimate interests and needs of the chronic mentally ill. The necessary clout is simply not there. Indeed, the cynic might be inclined to conclude that state government turns over commissioners as a way of avoiding the basic reforms that require both greater investment of funds and sustained attention to their effective management.

Local governments, although critical and important, are by necessity dependent on state resources. The political pitfalls just described have an effect on the ability of local government to deal independently with the needs of the chronic mentally ill. Despite this dependency, however, the role of local communities cannot be underestimated when it comes to housing, employment services, and development of therapeutic environments. All of these services are constrained by resource availability at the local government level. If the chronic mentally ill are to connect with the service system, it must occur at the local level. The role of local government as it relates to a number of legal issues will be addressed later. The point being emphasized here is that local government is more than an extension of the policies and resources emanating from federal and state governments. It is the milieu wherein citizen care and concern for the chronic mentally ill are either expressed by the provision of community-based services or fail to be expressed by such services.

The federal government, as previously mentioned, has avoided the chronic mentally ill. Even in the heyday of available federal funding for mental health services, no priority was given to serving the chronic mentally ill. Indeed, the federal reimbursement policy sought to entirely avoid this needy population. Priority during the deliberations that led to the enactment of the Community Mental Health Centers Act of 1963 was not the chronic client. The focus was on the mentally retarded and the acute mentally ill. It is fair to say that the "bold" approach of that time did not include the chronic mentally ill in any substantial way.

Subsequent developments at the federal level, although more specifically recognizing the needs of the chronic mentally ill, have been equally disappointing. The policy leadership and level of funding that many grew to expect from the federal government were lacking. The Carter initiatives, although commendable, were so broadly concerned with everybody's issues that by the time the Mental Health Systems Act became law, the Budget Reconciliation Act of 1981 easily blew it away. Generalized concern for cost containment and for a more limited federal government role eliminated the Mental Health Systems Act before it had a chance of being implemented. This, by the way, is a sobering example of how a strong upsurge of negative political sentiment can literally overturn several years of strenuous professional and constituency efforts to gain national recognition. The lesson here is that unless we are able to articulate national priorities and their rationale well enough, human service policies at the federal level are vulnerable. Among the populations that benefit from these policies, people like the chronic mentally ill who are least able to defend themselves will be the first casualties.

The federal response to other disabilities has been more successful. Multiple locations within the federal bureaucracy addressing the issues of the mentally retarded and developmentally disabled populations have created a broad constituency for meeting their service needs. The University Affiliated Facilities program for the developmentally disabled, for example, has generated enthusiastic involvement of the academic research and training community. The Medicaid Intermediate Care Facility for the Mentally Retarded program, by refinancing state institutional services to the mentally retarded, has had a profound effect on program philosophy, goals, and quality. The Protection and Advocacy program for the developmentally disabled is another example. Obviously, there has been no similar multipronged approach to meeting the needs of the chronic mentally ill at the federal or state levels. All the eggs have been placed in the basket of NIMH, an agency which itself has a history of isolation from other federal agencies and whose interests and resources have been directed to other concerns than the chronic mentally ill.

It is clear, in summary, that major obstacles to implementing programs for the chronic mentally ill exist at the federal, state, and local government levels. At the federal level, they include a poorly conceptualized role, the lack of priority, and too narrow a band of interest. At the state level, in addition to the lack of priority, there is little political and professional leadership and continuity. At the local level, there is no sustained independent role. Although dependent on state financial support and sanction, the local community is clearly the milieu in which programs succeed or fail. It is here that the chronic mentally ill person attains whatever quality of life is possible within the constraints of local government resources and capabilities.

FINANCIAL AND CONTROL ISSUES

The systems for financing services in both the private and public sectors do not relate realistically to the needs of the chronic mentally ill. The private practice model has already been identified as too narrow and restricted a service dimension. The matter of a multipronged approach to meeting needs has not been addressed. If anything, there is a dysfunctional quality to the reimbursement system that provides service coverage in the private sector. The recently developed diagnostic-related group (DRG) system of reimbursement seems likely to make financing of services to the chronic mentally ill even more inadequate. Although the DRG system has yet to encompass the chronic psychiatric population, one can anticipate applications that will lead to further restrictions on the already-limited days of reimbursable psychiatric services in private sector programs (6). Simply put, the name of the game is the rationing of services in order to contain costs with little regard for the consequences!

In the public sector, agency-designed budgets are also dysfunctional. To identify one agency as the single responsible authority, and to allocate funds to the line item that it represents in a federal, state, or local government budget misses the point of what the chronic mentally ill person needs. In truth, we have no mechanism for cutting across agency lines to allocate simultaneously a portion of their budgets to meeting such needs of the chronic mentally ill as income support, housing, social support, and clinical treatment. This has clearly been a problem for all three levels of government. The financing of single agencies, such as a department of mental health, to promote centralization and control over categorical funding streams results in more rather than less fragmentation of services.

Identifying the case manager role has been one way to orchestrate services to the chronic mentally ill at the community level. But case management fails when there are insufficient resources to go around. The maxim, "Nobody gives what he does not have," says it all! Attempts to coordinate resources at the administrative level of government where budgets are formulated have been singularly unsuccessful largely because of resource insufficiencies and the competition among constituencies. Agencies naturally acquire certain constituencies whom they "represent" in the budget formulation process. It is natural for these agencies to try to limit access to their resources to the "preferred customer," that is, their constituents, and to minimize spending on other clients. Thus, the very administrative structures that are created for the purposes of budgeting and control of expenditures stimulate competition and infighting among the health and human services organizations that have joint responsibility for meeting the needs of the chronic mentally ill. The history of the Title XX social services programs is illustrative of this dilemma. The Title XX program, generally, has not been very responsive to chronic mentally ill people even though deinstitutionalization is one of its highest priorities.

Aggravating an already problematic situation is the fact that mental health agencies are competing for a slice of the total state budget against much stronger constituencies, including interest groups for highway spending, liquor tax use, commerce and tourism, economic development, and the like. Politicians place higher value on meeting the needs of these interest groups than on the constituents of human service agencies. To the extent that the constituents of the human service agencies are consumed with infighting among themselves, they are correctly perceived as divided and weak—capable of being ignored with impunity.

Boggs (7), in reviewing the effects of the "cap" on federal spending for social services under Title XX of the Social Security Act, captures the weakness of human service providers as they struggle against one another for a larger share of a fixed budget:

> These days, almost any argument that a certain service (homemaker, chore services, case management, protective supervision, personal care, day care, to name a few) should be fundable under Title XX is immediately brushed off as irrelevant because service allocations within each state are to all intents and purposes frozen at the level in effect when that particular state reaches its cap on Federal spending.
>
> It is important for Federal policy makers to bear in mind that much of the pressure to find a way to use Title XX for health-related social and support services arises because the more appropriate resource for funding social services has been bottled up. Even the most elementary student of behavioral fisics knows that when you turn off the spigot at one point, more people line up to get more out of some other hydrant, drawing from the same underlying reservoir. (p 76)

Unfortunately, there is no solution in sight for this basic fact of economic and political life. As federal budget makers understand quite well, if they can limit growth of federal grant-in-aid and reimbursement programs, citizens will head for the state and local spigots to quench their thirst.

Under the circumstances, the only hope for the human service constituencies is for them to band together in a coalition that is stronger than
some of their non-human service competitors and go after a bigger slice
of the total state budget.

LEGAL ISSUES RELATED TO PROVIDING SERVICES

There is an inherent conflict in the law governing confinement for mental
illness, particularly chronic mental illness. It involves the balance between the individual's civil liberties and his need for help when mental
illness compromises his capacity to care for himself. A sense of the dilemma is conveyed by Teisher (8), a member of the California Alliance
for the Mentally Ill:

> It is, without any question, a civil libertarian's nightmare. Should we, in
> the name of liberty, ignore the truth about persistent, irrational behavior
> on the part of people whose judgment has deteriorated as a result of severe
> mental illness?
> Should we believe, as many civil liberties do, that mental illness has
> no impact on the ability of the psychotic to consider options and make choices
> and act effectively in his own behalf?
> Should we subscribe to the currently employed criteria for bringing
> mentally ill persons into involuntary treatment that being psychotic isn't
> enough? The victim of mental illness must be suicidal, homicidal, or in a
> state of advanced malnutrition to be considered for hospitalization?
> Over and over again we are confronted with human tragedy because
> mentally ill persons are granted their civil liberty even in the face of obvious
> mental disturbance. They are not stopped from committing heinous crimes,
> endangering neighborhoods, and putting themselves in mortal danger.
> These acts, on the part of a very few mentally disturbed individuals,
> do great harm to all mentally ill persons, who are "painted with the same
> brush," are damaged by the same cruel stigma.
> How very unfair to all gentle, loving mentally ill persons! How very
> short-sighted on the part of those advocates for freedom no matter what the
> consequences!
> Let's stop denying the reality and harshness of severe mental illness,
> and help before it is too late. (p 7)

This conflict obviously exacerbates the tension between the family
and the mentally ill person. The law has swung back and forth in its
emphasis on civil liberties and the need to exert social control. There is
evidence to suggest that the pendulum is swinging from the civil liber-
tarian view of the 1960s and early 1970s to a more conservative view in
the 1980s.

How are mental health services being affected by this tension and conflict? It is interesting to note that case law based on litigation such as *O'Connor v. Donaldson* (1975) (9) and *Wyatt v. Stickney* (1971) (10) have focused on patients in institutions. Only recently has litigation begun to deal with the consequences of community care of mentally ill persons (11). Interestingly, the cases involve liability for "wrongful discharge" and the "duty to warn" of mental health professionals, who are being held responsible for the injuries caused by former patients. The leading case in this regard is *Tarasoff v. Regents of the University of California* (1976) (12), which held that a therapist who knew that a patient threatened to harm a readily identifiable third party was required to warn that party of the possible danger.

Most states lack laws that specifically facilitate treatment and care of chronic mentally ill persons in the community. In addition, the laws do not adequately describe community and institutional services as parts of a continuum of care. In Virginia, for example, the state statute allows the court to select the least-restrictive environment for individuals who are being involuntarily committed to treatment. In point of fact, the court almost never decides in favor of the least-restrictive environment. When asked, judges say they would select the least-restrictive environment if they received assurances that placement in the community would offer the same level of control as an institution does. The courts do not take advantage of less-restrictive community program options because they lack the apparent level of control of an institution.

Some states, such as Wisconsin, allow the client to be committed to the local mental health service authority, which in turn assumes responsibility for the patient according to the court's prescription. This appears quite consistent with the professional view that a broad range of program options should be provided to chronic mentally ill people. As L.I. Stein (personal communication, 1985) reports, the Wisconsin community care model uses less-formal procedures to resolve problems instead of rushing to the court for a decision to convey the patient to a faraway state hospital. The model that Stein advocates results in the use of more community care options and a lower rate of state hospitalization.

During the last 25 years there has been considerable lag between enactment of laws that foster the practices advocated by mental health professionals and what actually takes place. Currently, many kinds of legislation are needed to assist the chronic mentally ill:

- Legislation to prevent discrimination in zoning, employment, insurance, and other areas.
- Laws to safeguard the rights of chronic mentally ill persons in the

community as well as in institutions under public and private control.

- Laws that promote easier, more rapid adjudication procedures where mental competency or partial competency is concerned—especially where there is need for rapid appointment of a guardian to act on behalf of the mentally incompetent person in situations which are urgent.
- Legislation at the local, state, and federal levels that clearly demonstrates society's commitment to treatment of chronic mentally ill persons in the environment that is least restrictive of personal liberty.
- Involuntary commitment legislation that emphasizes community support systems and that specifically authorizes involuntary treatment and care of reluctant mentally ill persons in a variety of outpatient settings such as psychosocial rehabilitation and/or residential programs.
- Legislative support for community mental health advocacy systems to help insure that the chronic patient's rights are respected.
- Legislation that specifically links institutional and community programs so that adequate predischarge planning and continuity of care takes place.

SOCIETAL STEREOTYPING AND ITS EFFECTS

Curtis (13), a respected authority on health and human services, gives voice to a myth that is widely held by laypersons and professionals alike: "The problems [associated with chronic mental illness] arise from a mental health care system that has failed repeatedly in the last 100 years to deliver on its promises to cure mental impairment." Suffice it to say, the cure standard of mental health service performance is an illusion that has reinforced a number of stereotypes about chronic mental illness. These include:

- Chronic mental illness is a static condition.
- Independent living is not feasible.
- "Normalization" of lifestyle is not achievable.
- Dangerousness is always associated with mental illness.
- The constitutional right to liberty and freedom cannot be handled by chronic mentally ill people.

These stereotypes embody an overly restrictive and pessimistic view of what the chronic mentally ill person can achieve in life.

There is need to counter these stereotypes with clear recognition of several points:

- Chronic mental illness is a continuing condition with numerous ups and downs and fluctuations in symptomatology and degree of functional limitations.
- There is need for others to view the treatment and care of each chronic mentally ill person in terms of improved functioning rather than cure with the goal of maintaining the individual at as high a functional level as possible in the context of the specific mental disorder.
- The chronic mentally ill person needs help with the basic necessities of living—shelter, food, clothing, transportation, and human support—all of which cannot be easily negotiated because of the individual's mental disorder.
- Interpersonal support and assistance from other people are needed as much by chronic mentally ill persons as by other people.

The remarkable success in improving the lives of mentally retarded persons in this country has come about through perseverance and consistency of actions, including development of national, state, and local organizations with consistent policy objectives; adherence to the clear ideology that mental retardation is not a disease; development of multipronged programs of education, habilitation, and residential care; consistent articulation of necessary legislation, programs, service standards, and funding levels at all levels of government; use of the courts to challenge all levels of government to do better; and acceptance of the reality of the disability while realizing that actions can be taken to mitigate its effects on individuals, families, and the community.

These actions on behalf of the mentally retarded have been taken by the professions, politicians, and persons from all strata of society. They are the prototype for broad-based, multilevel action for reform in any human service sector. The chronic mentally ill await the implementation of a similar multipronged aproach.

The way to deal with the problem of stereotyping in society is to broaden the base of citizen participation. Knowledgeable and informed constituencies must be formed. The relevant constituencies are consumers, service providers, advocates, and professional associations, to mention only the more obvious members. The direction and sustaining power of political influence is another important consideration. Any agency that is bereft of constituencies lacks power to compete for attention, resources, and legitimation.

Constituencies are the bridge between political, professional, and consumer interests. The constant tension involved in the competition for resources requires constant effort to reach consensus across constituencies. Most important is the achievement of consensus about the capacity that chronic mentally ill persons have to live lives of dignity and worth. The mental disorder is manageable and deserves the fullest professional attention.

NATIONAL POLICY IMPLICATIONS

The questions addressed in this chapter and the politics involved in implementing the approaches that work with the chronic mentally ill may be construed as state and local matters of no concern to the federal government. After all, the federal government has been able to avoid coverage of the 22- to 64-year-old adult population of mentally ill persons who reside in free-standing psychiatric facilities. Reinforcing this hands off policy is the fact that the federal government is running a deficit while many states at this time are enjoying surpluses. So why should the federal government become more involved than it is?

There are some reasons why national policies, even if low in cost and peripheral to the state and local action, make sense. To the extent that state and local governments have difficulty in asserting a priority for services to the chronic mentally ill, there is reason for national concern about an underserved, special-needs population whose civil rights and liberties may be jeopardized by the policies and practices of state and local governments.

Second, to the extent that educational institutions receive a variety of direct and indirect federal subsidies and do not turn out needed professionals for public sector service to the chronic mentally ill, there is reason for national concern about the consequences. Federal subsidies to educational institutions include direct student aid and guaranteed student loans. The federal government at marginal cost could earmark some of these subsidies for students of programs that teach the technologies that work for the chronic mentally ill. No new funds need be appropriated; existing student and guaranteed student loans would simply be set aside for students who chose to pursue undergraduate and graduate education majors in the departments and schools that teach the requisite course content. In this way, the pool of trained professionals would be enlarged and perhaps in the process come to realize that their guild interests should include the adequacy of funding for services to the chronic mentally ill.

There are rationales for extending existing federal programs to the chronic mentally ill. Chronic mental illness that develops prior to age 22 falls within the federal definition of "developmental disability" under the Developmental Disabilities Act of 1984 [Public Law 98-527, Sections 102(7)]. Strictly speaking, the chronic mentally ill are entitled to all the protections and services that flow from this important legislation. Advocates and the constituency of chronic mentally ill and their families can now press for greater attention and a fair share of available resources, including consideration at the federal and state levels for a share of the discretionary funds that are being directed to the Reagan Administration's supported work initiative.

NIMH has resources and a role to play in advocating and coordinating access to a range of federal program benefits, including income support under the Social Security Adult and Childhood Disability Insurance (SSDI) and Supplemental Security Income (SSI) programs, housing, employment services, vocational rehabilitation, special education, and the like. NIMH officials deserve credit for the role they played in the negotiations with the Social Security Administration that led to the proposed new medical criteria for assessing the eligibility of persons with mental disorders for SSDI and SSI. This is a low-cost role for NIMH that could be expanded. In time, such an advocacy and broker role could make a big difference.

NIMH also has research and training funds, some of which could be earmarked for projects that benefit the chronic mentally ill. Given the interest of the Reagan Administration in employment of persons with severe handicaps, where are the studies of the applicability of the supported work technology to the chronic mentally ill? If money is being spent to study the economics of mental health services, where is the project to document the short- and long-term benefits and costs of providing psychosocial rehabilitation in the community as an alternative to institutional care? Where are the replications of the benefit-cost analysis of the Wisconsin community care model that was published by Weisbrod et al. (15)? To our knowledge, only three studies even attempt to evaluate both the benefits and costs of care of the mentally ill in alternative settings (14–16). Of the three, only Weisbrod et al. employ an experimental design with random assignment of subjects into treatment and control groups (17).

Such applied research, if properly designed and conducted, is every bit as scientific as running rats or drug trials in laboratory settings. What is more, the economic payoff from applied studies may well be more immediate for all levels of government than that from the more basic investigations that are currently favored. The interests of society require attention not only to possible long-term payoffs but also to short-term benefits and costs. If state legislators and local officials shy away from immediate investments in community programs because they lack sufficient documentation of the benefits and costs, how can NIMH continue to abstain from funding scientific investigations to secure valid documentation?

The American Bar Association (ABA) periodically develops model laws relating to important legal issues which impact on all the states. ABA might well examine the specific areas identified above where legislation is needed to aid the chronic mentally ill. Again, national foundations and the Public Broadcasting System have a contribution to make in designing and implementing media campaigns to change the societal stereotypes of persons with chronic mental illness.

These are but a few illustrative ideas for national initiatives. Many more and perhaps better ideas could be generated if a strong stimulus at the national level were to get things moving. Let's face it, politics involves personalities, status, power, and influence. The constituencies court those who hold positions of power and influence, and those whom they court very often show reciprocity. It is no secret that the cause of the mentally retarded is aggressively and effectively argued by Mrs. Madeline Will, Assistant Secretary of the U.S. Department of Education. And there are those in the Reagan White House who listen.

There is nobody in Washington today who plays a similar role on behalf of the chronic mentally ill. As Mary Switzer, the great leader of the rehabilitation movement in the United States, knew and employed to good effect, legislators and executive branch officials whose families contain a handicapped member can be counted on to help out. They are willing and often eager to use their power and influence to secure needed research, training, and service programs. In the interplay of interests in the legislature, all legislators know that "everything is connected with everything."

So it is with politics and chronic mental illness. What is lacking is the necessary key federal legislator or executive branch official whose family member speaks to the importance of giving priority to the chronic mentally ill. When such leadership emerges, as in time it surely will, many ways will be found to accomplish what mental health professionals and constituencies now know can be done to improve the lives and functioning of persons with chronic mental illness.

REFERENCES

1. Musgrave RA, Musgrave PA: Public Finance in Theory and Practice. New York, McGraw-Hill, 1973
2. Mosher LR: Alternatives to psychiatric hospitalization: why has research failed to be translated into practice? N Eng J Med 309:1579–1580, 1983
3. Rubin A: Community Mental Health in the Social Work Curriculum. New York, Council on Social Work Education, 1979
4. Toward a National Plan for the Chronically Mentally Ill: Report to the Secretary by the Department of Health and Human Services

Steering Committee on the Chronically Mentally Ill (DHSS publication no. (ADM) 81-1077). Rockville, MD, Department of Health and Human Services, 1981

5. Lynn, LE Jr: The State and Human Services. Cambridge, MA, MIT Press, 1980
6. Evans RW: Health care technology and the inevitability of resource allocation and rationing decisions. JAMA 249:2047–2053, 1983
7. Boggs EM: Behavioral fisics, in Changing Government Policies for the Mentally Disabled. Edited by Bevilacqua JJ. Cambridge, MA, Ballinger, 1981
8. Teisher HG: The California Family State-Ment. Newsletter, Los Angeles, California Alliance for the Mentally Ill, June 1984
9. *O'Connor v. Donaldson.* 422 U.S. 563, 45 L.Ed. 2d 396, 95 S.Ct. 2486 (1975)
10. *Wyatt v. Stickney.* 325 F. Supp. 781 (M.D. Ala. 1971)
11. Rein WC: Having it both ways: surveying the area between least restrictive alternative and wrongful discharge. Mental Health and Mental Retardation Quarterly Digest 4(1):1, 22 March 1985
12. *Tarasoff v. Regents of the University of California.* 17 Cal. 3rd 425, 131 Cal. Rptr. 14, 551 p.2d 334 (1976), 83 A.L.R. 3rd 1166
13. Curtis WR: Deinstitutionalization in mental health care. Almanac. New York, New School for Social Research, February 1984
14. Murphy JG, Datel WE: A cost-benefit analysis of community versus institutional living. Hosp Community Psychiatry, 27:165–170, 1976
15. Weisbrod BA, Test MA, Stein LI: An Alternative to Mental Hospital Treatment. III. Economic Benefit-Cost Analysis. Madison, University of Wisconsin Press, 1978
16. Goldberg D, Jones R: The costs and benefits of psychiatric care. Unpublished report. Manchester, United Kingdom, Department of Psychiatry, University of Manchester, 1978
17. Noble JH Jr, Conley RW: Fact and conjecture in the policy of deinstitutionalization. Health Policy Quarterly 1:99–124, 1981

CHAPTER 7

The Role of Families in the Care of the Chronic Mentally Ill

SHIRLEY R. STARR

We are here today to address the issues which surround chronic mental illness. How did a conference of this magnitude encompass not only the opinions and perceptions of mental health professionals, but also the role of nonprofessionals? It would appear that we are reaching a stage of equity in planning and providing for the chronic mentally ill—professionals and nonprofessionals sharing the job of disseminating knowledge and influencing and helping to determine social policy affecting this group. When did this all begin? What are the factors that promoted this phenomenon?

The legitimatizing of self-help groups during the past decade is certainly an important factor. The history of the self-help movement is an interesting one. While the concept of self-help is not a new phenomenon, a recognized legitimate role for self-help groups is relatively new. There are two major reasons for this: 1) Such groups have grown enormously, and they have succeeded in developing a sophisticated understanding of the specific systems and the political process. 2) The interest in self-help activities has increased as a direct result of economic and political changes in our society during this past decade. Shortages of national resources and a myriad of economic ills have proved intractable to fiscal and monetary policy. The entire question of whether the federal government should be the agent of first resort with respect to social and health care is presently being debated, and a presidential candidate was elected on a platform which said "No" to that question. With the reduction in social and health programs during the past four years, professional providers and

149

state mental health systems have directed their attention to the role that voluntary organizations can play in redressing the effect of cuts in services to the mentally ill.

A number of hypotheses have been advanced to explain the origins and growth of voluntary associations. The classic statement of the late Professor Louis Wirth of the University of Chicago School of Sociology (1) still offers insight into the origin. He wrote:

Urban life is characterized by the substitution of secondary for primary contacts, the weakening of bonds of kinship, and the declining social significance of the family, the disappearance and the undermining of the traditional basis of social solidarity.

Being reduced to a stage of virtual impotence as an individual the urbanite is bound to exert himself by joining with others of similar interest into organized groups to obtain his ends . . .

Katz and Bender (2) in a more contemporary explanation of the origins of the self-help movement wrote:

When people feel themselves abandoned or frustrated by conventional society, they can sometimes bypass established institutions and create informal organizations on the side. To the extent that a voluntary association has a "mission" it can be referred to as a social movement.

Such grass-roots movements serve to provide otherwise unavailable services, to protest indignities, to escape suffering, to relieve tension, to explain confusing events or in some way to create a more tolerable way of life than is afforded by existing formal organizations.

Irving Zola (3) points to the way self-help groups have grown up around those people who were abandoned by the helping professions either because they represented its failures or because they had socially unacceptable problems. All such explanations have in common the theme of disillusionment with established helping services.

In mental health, these feelings were exacerbated by the presumptive belief of many early psychiatrists in the theory of "family as cause" and by the practice of excluding families from a collaborative effort with the psychiatrist in caring for the mentally ill relative. So families began to read books to seek the information they needed and began to find others with whom they could share common experiences and learn from one another how to handle the challenges of chronic mental illness. Somehow, the process of seeing that other people also struggle with similar problems helps to sustain an individual. A successful experience not only helps morale, but it offers another option to a family looking for some success. That has been the experience of those groups that were formed locally in response to local conditions in state mental health systems and eventually came together to begin The National Alliance for the Mentally Ill.

In September 1979, under the aegis of the University of Wisconsin at Madison, more than 200 persons from many states attended a conference on "Forming a National Network." Two days later, at the end of the conference, these individuals returned to their respective localities to seek agreement from their local groups to join such an alliance. Approval from the majority of these groups was forthcoming within the month. With a treasury of somewhat more than $3,000 donated by the conference attendees, an office was opened in Washington, D.C., in January 1980, manned by one volunteer. Within months, a major foundation recognized the importance of this movement and the cause it served and provided a large three-year grant to insure its continuance. From such modest beginnings, The National Alliance for the Mentally Ill now encompasses affiliates in all 50 states, with a membership of 30,000 families.

However, it was not a simple matter to get from September 1980 to this conference today. Our arrival on the scene was met with mixed responses. Self-help has only recently been recognized as a significant force in the human services area. Not only did professional organizations view us with some concern, so did the preexisting mental health advocacy groups. Both worried about the displacement effect and our competence. The National Alliance affiliates worried about neither. They believed that self-help groups did not need to be in competition with the professionals and with other advocacy groups. They believed that they offered a means of implementing programs that could promote the well-being of the mentally ill in the community, and they believed that they could provide essential information and support to the mental health professionals. They recognized the inherent antagonism toward their self-help efforts because of the challenge they posed to the existing order.

However, the existing order was what this national organization wanted to alter. They recognized also that they could easily be manipulated into becoming responsible for problems and services that are beyond individual control and, further, be used to absolve those in power of responsibility for dealing with the many problems. A clear agenda, even in its early days, characterized the National Alliance for the Mentally Ill. The inherent political potential of this organization was the best insurance against being manipulated and against the state and federal bureaucracies abrogating their responsibilities. The agenda of the National Alliance called for national government support for the care of the mentally ill and for support of those programs that needed to be available; the same is now being asked of state bureaucracies.

The concern of the professional groups and other advocacy organizations was mirrored in the concern the family self-help movement in mental health felt toward professionals. The movement began (as many grass roots groups begin) with a strong streak of antiprofessionalism. Some of that has been ameliorated through five years of cooperative ventures in four years of lean times. During the past five years, we have appeared at hundreds of professional conferences and spoken to thousands of professionals and thousands of families and ex-patients. Today we are here speaking on "The Role of Families." That was the basis for the formation of The National Alliance for the Mentally Ill—the founders believed there was a role for families.

The consistent view of those who work with families is that it matters not what you call them—self-help, mutual aid, support systems—they are the fastest growing component of the human service industry. Nor is it surprising. Man is a social animal who throughout his history has banded together for problem solving and survival (4).

The problems we face today, six years after the first Conference on the Chronic Mental Patient, are indeed complex. In 1978, the conference identified these issues as being of primary importance: deinstitutionalization; funding for chronic mental patients; suitable training for psychiatrists in caring for chronic mental patients; low status accorded chronic mental patients by psychiatrists; the need for a continuum of community care facilities; and adequate housing, job opportunities, and rehabilitation services. Today, the same issues demand our attention. Moreover, they exist in a social climate far less benign than in 1978 and are, therefore, more difficult to resolve. They are exacerbated by an environment within which social policy decisions are made that profoundly and adversely affect the chronic mentally ill.

If we look at deinstitutionalization, we see that its effects remain— replaced in many states by the term "deflection." "Deflection" is a blatant description of a policy that keeps many chronic patients from entering a state hospital and, if admitted, encourages premature discharge into a community ill prepared to provide for them and hostile to having them. As much as any one single factor, deinstitutionalization has caused the presence of so many of the chronic mentally ill among the homeless that we witness these days.

An examination of today's funding policies reveals that the chronic mentally ill have been affected by federal cuts in research and training funds and by drastic cuts in entitlement programs. These are the programs that provide the generic services needed by all human beings but that are most difficult to obtain by a handicapped constituency. Finally, funding cuts have also greatly reduced the quality of care in existing programs and all but eliminated many new programs.

While funding for research has fared the best in these worst of all times, the level of funding for an illness that is so pervasive and, in its most serious form, so disabling, is a disgrace. Funding for research in mental illness has not kept pace with the cost of living and, measured in real buying power, has fallen far behind. The hope for cures diminishes with each annual National Institute of Mental Health (NIMH) budget. Compared to the federal commitment to other areas of the budget—the cost of one B1 bomber equals the entire yearly budget of NIMH—the mental health of this nation has a very low priority.

The lack of suitable training for psychiatrists to care for the chronic mentally ill and the low status accorded chronic mentally ill patients by psychiatrists are both functions of inadequate investment in the mental health care delivery system. Were there incentives for treating the chronic patient, status might accrue to those psychiatrists accepting them as patients. Reimbursement could be made comparable to or better than that received by those who limit their practice to nonpsychotic patients. Why shouldn't there be incentives to treating the more difficult patient? Isn't this the population that most taxes the public pocketbook by using acute and emergency services in unexpected proportions? Cost-benefit analysis could make an excellent case for financial incentives in terms of benefit to patients, psychiatrists, and the public.

Six years after the first Conference on the Chronic Mental Patient, we must admit that the problems have not gone away. The continuing prevalence of high-risk populations in a time of reduced investment means that the problems will most likely continue.

What is the role of families—the non-mental health professionals—in providing care and support for the chronic mentally ill clients? In every community a wide range of services is needed. Helpers are needed unless the professionals have shared the same experience as the client and/or the family. Obviously, such shared experience is not possible, nor is it even always desirable. There are other equally important criteria for becoming a mental health professional. But without that shared experience, full understanding is absent. What families share with one another and what clients share with one another is the knowledge derived from the existential experience of enduring the ravages of a puzzling illness. For the family, that means witnessing the decline of a loved one and the laying aside of their appropriate expectations for that individual. It has also meant for them the frustration of seeking solutions to the problems that accompany such an illness and finding institutions resistant to change and practitioners unsympathetic to the family's situation. For the individual with mental illness, we can only begin to imagine what that means. Certainly the experience of mental patients provides for them the highest degree of legitimacy in their roles as advocates. To the extent that they are able to articulate their perceptions and overcome the constraints of a communicative disorder, they are—without exception—the ultimate consumer and advocate.

There is a long history of parents' activism on behalf of their children to relieve the children's suffering and to insure their rights. Historically, these were parents who found the traditional institutions lacking in their response and resistant to change. Parents advocated on behalf of better schools, better health care, and better opportunities for their children. The family self-help movement in mental health is a relatively new entry in the field. Its mandate provides the answer to "What is the role of families?"

1. To provide support to families in dealing with mental illness in a family.
2. To bring about change in the institutions that serve their relatives.
3. To protect and care about the mentally ill.
4. To support the search for cures.

Family Support

The backbone of the family self-help movement is family support. All affiliates of The National Alliance for the Mentally Ill provide family support to their members through regular support groups. These support groups are usually facilitated by a skilled (and compassionate) family member or sometimes by a similar professional. Families join together to speak with one another on ways in which to cope and to learn skills in locating needed resources and advocating on behalf of their family member. A unifying theme is the ways in which parents have been made to feel incompetent or culpable. The support group offers the place where their experience can be understood, where their anger can be given some legitimacy, and where they can receive concrete help. Inevitably, family support groups come to the realization that more needs to be done than expressing and sharing frustration. That realization usually translates into action directed toward institutional change. That is the beginning of the end of powerlessness.

Bringing About Change

While that realization may be the beginning of the end of powerlessness, changing the system is not all that simple. The action most groups take is a form of confrontation of those powerful institutions that serve their relatives. Real systemic change is a long time in coming, and confrontations are often painful. Staying power is needed, and families under stress do not always have that staying power. However, one of the distinguishing characteristics of the self-help movement has been the emergence of leaders, usually only a few and sometimes only one. But when the energies of these visionaries flag or turn to other activities, others have appeared to take up the gauntlet. It is estimated in studies of the self-help movement that a group can accomplish extraordinary things with only 10 percent of the group in positions of top leadership and another 25 percent as committed and working members.

Advocacy groups use different strategies to bring about fundamental change. Many use several strategies at one time. Whatever strategy or strategies a group chooses, however, the critical first step is acquiring the basic facts about the institutions they want to confront. Where does the institution get its funds? Is it a public institution or a private one or a quasi-governmental agency? Who are the people in charge? What are their positions? What is their reputation? What are the rules and regulations that act as constraints upon the institution? Once these facts have been ascertained, the weaknesses and vulnerabilities in the system are revealed and the strategies can be chosen. The first requirement for a good advocate is being an informed one.

Networking with other groups who share the common problem or those whose participation will strengthen the potential of both groups to effect change is a useful strategy. A coalition with professional groups is frequently utilized on the basis that both groups would benefit from an improved mental health system or institution.

The introduction of needed legislation is an important tool in the mental health advocate's kit. Groups with family members who are lawyers have a distinct advantage over those who do not. Litigation is usually seen as an act of last resort because of its costly nature and the protracted nature of the judicial process. Sometimes, however, it is the only way in which to effect change. When successful, it is one of the heady victories that spur self-help groups on to continue their advocacy efforts.

An extraordinary characteristic of the self-help movement and one that needs to be acknowledged is the transition of the members from a position of self-interest to a raised consciousness of the rights and interests of the whole class of mentally ill persons and to action on behalf of that class. This characteristic is most poignantly demonstrated when one observes the work and dedication of family members whose relatives are no longer living. Altruism within a self-help group is a certain indicator of the enormous growth of that group.

Providing Care and Support for the Mentally Ill

Families, to the extent they are able, provide care for their mentally ill relative. But for many chronic patients, families no longer exist. Parents of older chronic patients have either died or are so aged and disabled themselves that they can no longer provide support or care for the seriously ill family member. When families have not dispersed, care and support is often shared by siblings. When families no longer live in the same locality, there are real problems. Which sibling? Which area? Maintaining contact with a chronic patient via the mails or by telephone is often difficult because of the temporary nature of chronic patients' housing arrangements. Too often contact is broken for months and years at a time. Sometimes this is at the patient's initiative.

Even when parents are still alive and financially able to support their mentally ill relative, it is not always the most appropriate choice to have an adult son or daughter living at home. That is why housing has been identified as the number 1 need in a National Alliance for the Mentally Ill affiliate survey in a major city (5). That is also why many groups involve themselves in pressuring state agencies for additional funds for housing, in creating programs under their own aegis, or joining with social agencies that traditionally provide this service. For some groups, the inherent conflict between being a provider and an advocate proves to be untenable. Other groups successfully manage that conflict by creating separate corporations for provision of services. The important thing to emphasize here is the ability of the family self-help movement to respond to what is lacking in the system. That response is always to supply it themselves or to see that it is supplied.

Caring for mentally ill relatives after parents are dead is the common concern of all parents of the mentally ill (and other handicapped groups). Most families lack the necessary financial resources to adequately assure good care for their mentally ill relative. Without assurances that the federal government will continue entitlement programs to the mentally disabled, families struggle with what John Pringle, the English founder of The Schizophrenia Foundation, has called the "After I'm Gone Syndrome."

A new development in the family self-help movement for the mentally ill is the emergence of services designed to meet that need. Some of the shortcomings of the programs being advanced are obviously of a financial nature. What can be done without pricing the programs out of the reach of many families? PACT, a not-for-profit agency in Chicago, Illinois, is a prototype for this type of agency response to the problem. PACT is struggling with the financial aspects of provision of needed guardianship services and is seeking nontraditional methods of funding such services. Parent advocates sit on the board, were active in its inception, and have been advisers to the professional staff on what kind of provisions are needed. PACT is attempting to offer a kind of caring beyond death. Whether it is possible for any but the wealthier families to provide this service remains to be seen. But it is an attempt to provide humane, caring individuals to maintain contact with the chronic patient after the family is gone.

Supporting the Search for Cures

Advocacy also involves exerting pressure on the executive and legislative branches of the federal government to make a commitment to research in mental illness comparable to the ones it has made to heart disease and cancer, for example. It involves also convincing foundations to underwrite mental illness research because of the contribution the foundation can make to finding a cure. State and local governments cannot fund this undertaking. Only the federal government and some large foundations have that kind of capability. Advocates need to undertake a massive and ongoing national fund-raising effort to get the funds needed to achieve significant breakthroughs. Such a fund-raising effort requires a massive public education program aimed at changing public attitudes about mental illness—attitudes that reflect the public view of mental illness as social deviation and that do not recognize mental illness as illness. Giving money to research efforts is a widely respected tradition. Mental illness has to be seen as part of that tradition. To stimulate a response from the public, the National Alliance for the Mentally Ill has created a foundation for that purpose. It is seeking other national mental health groups to join in this effort. The same kind of strategies that have been utilized in other advocacy efforts of this movement are being called upon. All of the skills learned through earlier battles will be utilized. The same dedication will need to be demonstrated. The future is uncertain, but this is a beginning, and it is one of the most important roles that the family self-help movement can assume.

REFERENCES

1. Wirth L: Urbanism as a Way of Life. Chicago, University of Chicago Press, 1964
2. Katz AH, Bender EI: The Strength in Us. Indianapolis, New Viewpoints, 1976

3. Zola I: Helping One Another: A Brief History of Mutual Aid Groups. Waltham, MA, Brandeis University, 1975 (mimeographed)
4. Demone HW Jr: Introduction, in Directory of Mutual Help Organizations in Massachusetts, 4th ed. Blue Cross and Blue Shield, 1974
5. Alliance for the Mentally Ill of Greater Chicago: Inventory of Family Needs, 1981

CHAPTER 8

Severely Emotionally Disturbed Children and Adolescents

IRA S. LOURIE, M.D.
JUDITH KATZ-LEAVY, M.ED.

The labeling of children and adolescents as chronically mentally ill is not within the traditions of the child mental health movement. The nature of this movement is alien to the concepts of chronicity and rehabilitation. Favored instead are the concepts of continual growth leading to habilitation. Nonetheless, children and adolescents with long-term, or "chronic," needs have long been recognized.

To avoid the negative connotations of the chronic concept, terminology that better suits the description of these children and adolescents should be used. Chronic or long-term emotional problems are best viewed as severe disturbances in growth requiring extra help in habilitation. "Severely emotionally disturbed" is the term most widely used to describe this population. While it avoids describing a hopeless condition, it conveys the seriousness of the condition and the high degree of service that these children require. This term also has the advantage of being the concept in current use within the special education system.

These young people require a wide range of services that may include long-term out-of-home placement as well as community-based, family-oriented care. Many of these children are presently lost to adequate treatment because appropriate services are lacking or because they are misplaced in child welfare and juvenile justice programs, where their mental health problems have not been recognized. Knitzer (1) reported that two-thirds, or 2,000,000, of these children are not receiving needed services, and many of the children in facilities are receiving inappropriate care.

ISSUES OF DEFINITION

The definition of the severely emotionally disturbed population has long been of issue. While there has been a reluctance to call the population chronically mentally ill, it is also clear that another definition has not been easily forthcoming. The term "severely emotionally disturbed" has been borrowed from education, but a formal, generally accepted definition has not yet been developed. Until the time that the concept is defined, research and service planning will be hampered.

Crucial to being able to define this population in a meaningful light is the development of language that cuts across the many disciplines represented in the multiagency service network. Until that time when professionals in various agencies use common definitions and diagnostic labels to identify and describe this population, coordinated service delivery will lag. A common language will allow for better coordination and service delivery. The several historic attempts to define the population are reported in this section.

In 1970 the Joint Commission on the Mental Health of Children (2) defined a broad category of emotionally disturbed child:

> one whose progressive personality development is interfered with or arrested by a variety of factors so that he shows an impairment in the capacity expected of him for his age and endowment: (1) for reasonably accurate perception of the world around him; (2) for impulse control; (3) for satisfying and satisfactory relations with others; (4) for learning; or (5) for any combination of these. (p 253)

This definition set the stage for later ones by focusing on the role of developmental tasks and ability to function at an age-appropriate level as the major factors.

To add the concept of severity to this definition is not very difficult. Since the basic parameter of the definition is disability, the degree of disability then becomes the parameter by which seriousness or severity is defined. Severity can also be related to length of disability, so that the long-term nature of a child's problem could define him or her as severely emotionally disturbed.

A child and adolescent definition was developed in 1980 by the National Institute of Mental Health (NIMH) for the National Plan for the Chronically Mentally Ill (3). Although the definition was of chronic mental illness, the terms and issues presented fit equally well for the severely emotionally disturbed. This definition was developed to be used for improving service delivery to these children. It was a working definition that had an individualized treatment plan for each child as an end product; this plan and the accompanying definition take into consideration the individual's degree of disability and the appropriate specific service needs of that youngster and his or her family. Diagnostic labels alone cannot be used to plan for this population. As with adults, a diagnostic label does not specify the severity or chronicity of the disability and does not correlate with treatment requirements. A child or adolescent with almost any diagnostic level may require long-term, highly structured, and supervised care. Therefore, this definition was based on disability, with diagnosis, duration, and response to treatment being modifying criteria (see Table 1).

The 1980 definition has been the basis of many discussions about the most valid definition of severely emotionally disturbed children and adolescents. This discussion came to a peak in the 1983 workshop jointly sponsored by the National Institute of Mental Health and the State Mental Health Representatives for Children and Youth of the State Mental Health Program Directors. The conclusion of this panel was to use a definition similar to NIMH's 1980 definition and to hold to the following guidelines:

> There is a need for a diagnostic scheme that has more relevance [than the *Diagnostic and Statistical Manual of Mental Disorders (Third Edition) (DSM-III)*] for treatment and resource planning purposes. There is also a need to develop a definition and diagnostic process that can be understood and utilized by all agencies serving children. Therefore, *it is suggested that a definition based on some categorization of social functioning be adopted.*
> *A definition [should be developed] for the types of children to be targeted.* Such a definition is needed for several reasons, including:
> (a) the need for a common language across child service and management agencies:
> (b) the need to tie diagnosis more closely to actual services;
> (c) the development of system-wide plans;
> (d) the development of individual treatment plans;
> (e) the desire to improve epidemiological information and statistical data;
> (f) eligibility to receive services in many states;
> (g) research purposes; and
> (h) funding purposes, especially under Medicaid, SSI and other entitlement and insurance programs.
> The parameters suggested [for such a definition] are:
> (a) *The population selected should have a multiagency need* (must be involved in more than just one system);
> (b) *Assessment should be based on some type of social functioning categorization rather than diagnosis;*
> (c) *Children to be included . . . must have a mental health defined problem* (i.e., fit one of the diagnoses included in *DSM-III*).

Although it is clear that there is no conclusion as to how either chronic mental illness or serious emotional disturbance in children and

Table 1.　Definition of Chronic Mental Illness in Children and Adolescents Developed by the National Institute of Mental Health in 1980

1. *Disability.* The term "chronically mentally ill child or adolescent" is defined to refer to a person under the age of 18 with a severe chronic disability which:
 (a) represents an emotional and/or organic impairment, which is manifest by emotional or behavioral symptoms, that is not *solely* a result of mental retardation or other developmental disabilities, epilepsy, drug abuse or alcoholism; and,
  (1) continues for more than one year, or on the basis of specific diagnosis is *likely* to continue for more than one year; and,
  (2) results in substantial functional limitations of major life activities in two or more of the following areas:
   a. self-care at an appropriate developmental level,
   b. perceptive and expressive language,
   c. learning,
   d. self-direction, including behavioral controls, decision making, judgment and value systems,
   e. capacity for living in a family or family equivalent,
 (b) reflects the person's need for a combination and sequence of special, interdisciplinary or generic care, treatment, or other services which are of extended duration and are individually planned and coordinated.

2. *Diagnosis.* Although, as stated before, diagnosis cannot be used as a basis for defining chronic mental illness, certain diagnostic categories (as defined in *DSM-III*) are most often associated with it. They are:

A. *Pervasive developmental disorders*
This category includes autism and later-onset developmental disorder. It is associated with lack of responsiveness to other people, deficits in language development, peculiar speech patterns, bizarre responses to the environment.

B. *Childhood schizophrenia*
Pervasive developmental disorders accompanied by second order schizophrenic symptoms such as delusions, hallucinations, incoherence, or marked loosening of associations. This group is considered as part of the schizophrenias by *DSM-III*. This category also includes mentally retarded children who demonstrate psychotic symptoms.

C. *Schizophrenia of adult-type manifesting in adolescence*
Many schizophrenias first appear during adolescence. These are identical to adult syndromes and are not associated with severe pervasive developmental delays seen in childhood schizophrenia.

D. *Severe behavioral disorders requiring long-term residential care*
These disorders are classified in *DSM-III* as conduct disorders of various types. For inclusion in this definition they must be so severe as to be associated with a degree of disability whose treatment requires 24-hour care and supervision.

Table 1. continued

E. *Mental retardation and other developmental disabilities with accompanying mental disorders*
Behavioral and/or psychotic symptoms are complications which can determine how well an otherwise developmentally disabled child or adolescent can function. Concurrent behavioral or psychotic problems are the only reason that many developmentally disabled persons require inpatient or other sheltered care.

F. *Other disorders*
Any childhood disorder which on a case-by-case basis fully fills the disability and duration requirements of this definition, such as affective disorders and certain disorders with severe medical implications (anorexia nervosa and ulcerative colitis).

3. *Duration.* As stated in the definition, the disability must have continued for more than one year, or, on the basis of a specific diagnosis, is likely to continue for more than one year. Childhood schizophrenia and autism are examples of such diagnoses. These diagnoses suggest a prognosis of long-term service need, minimally several years, with a large percentage (at least 50 to 80%) requiring care into adult life. All such children under 12 with diagnoses which indicate such prognosis should be included in the group of chronically mentally ill. While it is true that some childhood schizophrenics have isolated psychotic episodes without long-term care needs, this group is very small and the needs of these children should be dealt with individually [4, 5].

Youth whose schizophrenic symptoms and related disability manifest between 12 and 18 years of age usually do so with more adult like symptoms. However, their course and prognosis is often similar to that of children (especially with younger adolescents) and they usually require long-term services. Although some acute schizophrenic episodes in adolescents prove to be short-term, with chronicity not becoming an issue, the need for a full range of services is still necessary.

4. *Response to treatment.* Chronicity of mental health problems is often related to the availability of treatment. A condition should not be considered chronic until it has proven unresponsive to appropriate treatment modalities of sufficient intensity, or on the basis of diagnosis is likely to prove unresponsive. As with duration, the determination of likelihood will be made on the basis of the same specific diagnosis. However, responsiveness to treatment is much more difficult to predict than duration and untreated or inadequately treated children should only be classified as chronic with great caution.

adolescents should be defined, there is a growing consensus as to the issues which need to be included in such a definition. The development of the Child and Adolescent Service System Program (CASSP) by the NIMH in 1984 (see page 179) used this prevailing thought to come up with its definition. The CASSP definition had five criteria, which were written broadly so that states could redefine the population to meet local needs.

Age is the first CASSP criterion. It is significant that even the age at which an individual is no longer a child or adolescent is a criterion on which there is no consensus. The final determinations are usually political in nature and focus on an age up to either 18 or 21 years.

Disability is the second and most important criterion. The greatest degree of consensus is in this area. Definition is felt by most to require a primary focus on the child's degree of disability. CASSP said that the degree of ability to perform in the family, in school, and in the community is the basic issue which determines the need for CASSP services.

Multiagency need is the third CASSP criterion. By definition a severely emotionally disturbed child or adolescent should have a degree of disturbance that requires services from at least two community service agencies, such as mental health, health, special education, juvenile justice, or social welfare.

Mental illness is the fourth CASSP criterion. Although there was no consensus that *DSM-III* (6) served a useful role in classifying mental illness, it is self-evident that being "mentally ill" or "emotionally disturbed" (either chronically or severely) requires the presence of a mental illness as defined by *some* classification.

Duration is the last CASSP criterion. The constant growth and change capacity represented in the process of child development makes a long-term assessment of the child's problem mandatory before a classification of chronically or severely disturbed can be assigned. Therefore, at least a one-year duration of the disability is the suggested limit, with the exception of those conditions (such as childhood psychosis) in which there is a substantial risk of duration over one year.

This CASSP definition unfortunately represents the state of the art. Further research and clinical review will be necessary before a more useful definition can be devised. Until that time scientific, clinical, and system-building efforts will be hampered and definitions used will be subject to political interpretation.

NUMBERS OF SEVERELY EMOTIONALLY DISTURBED CHILDREN

The lack of consensus regarding a definition of the severely emotionally disturbed child and adolescent population, as described above, results in a parallel lack of agreement in developing a national data base on this population. Estimates of numbers of children with mental disorders of sufficient severity and duration to be considered chronic range from very narrow interpretations (such as the estimate in the 1980 National Plan) (3) to broader interpretations (such as those presented by Knitzer (1) and Gilmore et al. (7).

The Department of Health and Human Services Steering Committee on the Chronically Mentally Ill (8) used a standard for defining chronicity in adults of an uninterrupted psychiatric hospitalization of 90 days or more. Although this figure does not include a proportion of the chronic mentally ill persons in the community, it does represent a fair estimate of the scope of the adult chronic mentally ill population. Lourie et al. (3) clearly demonstrate that this model does not work well with children and adolescents. There are there reasons for this. The first is that many children are hospitalized for over 90 days even though their level of disability would not classify them as chronically mentally ill. For some children an extended hospital stay reflects a situation in which appropriate family or community resources are not available. (While many adults who could be deinstitutionalized also remain in hospitals because appropriate community resources are not available, they still fit into the category of the chronic mentally ill on the basis of disability.) Second, many of the most severely disturbed autistic and psychotic children are never hospitalized either because family and community services are appropriate and available or because proper hospital resources are not available. The third issue is that residential care of over 90 days can, at times, be the most appropriate treatment for certain children and adolescents with less severe, nonchronic problems.

For purposes of developing a service model for chronic mentally ill children and adolescents, Lourie et al. (3, p 8) used an estimate of 70,000. This figure encompasses the 50,000 children and adolescents estimated by the NIMH Division of Biometry and Epidemiology to have been hospitalized or placed in a mental health residential treatment setting for over 90 days in 1980, the 10,000 estimated nonhospitalized autistic and schizophrenic children and the 10,000 mentally retarded children and adolescents with long-term severe emotional disorders. Lourie et al. (3, p 9) did, however, acknowledge that uncounted behaviorally disordered children with severe chronic emotional problems housed in non-mental health settings may number from 400,000 to 800,000.

Knitzer (1) reported that there are approximately 3,000,000 severely mentally disturbed children and adolescents in the United States today. Gilmore et al. (7) concluded that the most appropriate figure for estimating the need for mental health services among children and adolescents is a figure of 11.8 percent of the under-18 population presented by

Gould et al. (9). When this figure is applied to 1980 U.S. Census figures (10), an estimated 7,500,000 individuals under the age of 18 are in need of mental health services. This estimate was actually quite similar to that of the Joint Congressional Commission on Mental Illness and Mental Health (11), which used a figure of 10 percent of the population of all ages as in need of mental health services. This estimate, generally accepted as a conservative estimate of need, was based on input from a variety of sources, including surveys of 11 different communities from 1916 to 1958. The 11.8 percent figure of Gould et al. is also similar to that of the more recent President's Commission on Mental Health (12), which estimated that 5 to 15 percent of the 3- to 15-year-old cohort were in need of mental health services. Based on the study of Robins (13), the commission came to the opinion that the 15 percent figure was the most realistic estimate.

In their paper, Gilmore et al. (7) further attempted to estimate the prevalence of specific functional deficit clusters appearing in mentally ill children and adolescents by applying the 11.8 percent figure of Gould et al. to the epidemiological studies of Rutter et al. (14). Using this procedure, Gilmore et al. estimated that children with psychosis (excluding autism) constitute 0.23 percent of the total population under 18 years of age. When applied to the 1980 census, this results in an estimate of 146,000 psychotic children and adolescents. Similarly, 4.5 percent (2,869,000) of the total child and adolescent population is estimated to have anxiety/affective disorders; 3.5 percent (2,231,000) have conduct disorders, and 1.1 percent (701,000) are multiply handicapped. These estimates total 5,957,000 seriously affected children and adolescents.

Gilmore et al. also describe a population of children at risk of functional impairment because of demographic factors frequently associated with mental illness, such as:

a) failure in infancy and early development to secure basic nurturance necessary to achieve security, identity, and self-worth; b) environmental stresses that precipitate social breakdown; c) families who have experienced mental illness; d) children and adolescents who have been subject to child abuse, neglect, or sexual abuse; and e) children and adolescents suffering chronic physical illness to such an extreme that mental illness may be precipitated. (7)

Lieberman (15) estimates that this "at-risk" group constitutes 2 to 12 percent of the population (both children and adults). While this group certainly needs to be included in developing any comprehensive plan for mental health services, the actual figures have not been computed for inclusion in this chapter because the authors feel that an at-risk group does not fit any of the definitions of chronic or severe emotional disability.

While an exact figure for the number of severely emotionally disturbed children and adolescents in the United States obviously does not exist, it is also clear that the original National Plan 1980 estimate of 70,000 is far too low and ignores a large number of severely emotionally disturbed children and adolescents with problems of long-term or recurring duration. For purposes of service system planning, CASSP has utilized Knitzer's (1) figure of 3,000,000. Although this figure could also turn out to be an underestimate (as suggested by Gilmore et al. [7]), CASSP believes it is a useful and conservative estimate which can, at least, serve as the beginning point for improved data collection and service system planning.

SERVICES FOR SEVERELY EMOTIONALLY DISTURBED CHILDREN AND ADOLESCENTS: COMMUNITY, STATE, AND FEDERAL CONSIDERATIONS

Community-Level Services

The service system described in this chapter[1] is not new in concept or particularly innovative. It is based on the principles elucidated in the 1969 Report of the Joint Commission on the Mental Health of Children (2) and is reflected in Public Law 94-142, The Education for All Handicapped Children Act. It is described in the options paper prepared for the Select Panel for the Promotion of Child Health (16). The President's Commission on Mental Health (12), along with the Mental Health Systems Act, Public Law 96-398, encourages development of such coordinated systems of care. NIMH's Most in Need program funded such demonstration programs in several Native American communities. While this spirit is present and the technology is available, this system for the care of severely emotionally disturbed children and adolescents has not been universally or even widely implemented.

---

[1]The section on community-level services is taken with minor changes from the chapter "Chronically Mentally Ill Children and Adolescents," in the *National Plan for the Chronically Mentally Ill* (3). Much of the information was derived from Silver's (16) Options Paper prepared for the Select Congressional Panel for the Promotion of Child Health.

Services for severely emotionally disturbed children and adolescents need to be comprehensive enough to provide for the needs of a wide range of long-term, severe disabilities. A continuum of care must be provided in which each individual child can obtain the level and type of services needed at any one time. The components of such a system must include family and community-based resources as well as acute, intermediate, and long-term 24-hour programs. A principle basic to this service continuum is that an individual's needs are expected to change as he or she develops and as his or her family changes. This may be reflected in either steady predictable growth or in rapid unpredictable fluctuations, both of which may require related changes in those services needed.

The primary link between the continuum of services and the child or adolescent is the family. The parents or guardians have primary responsibility for initiating services and must participate in the planning for their provision. Ideally, the parents have ultimate control over what services are sought and accepted. There are exceptions, such as when a court removes such controls from a family. Parents have differing abilities to accept and live with the symptoms of a severely emotionally disturbed child or adolescent. Some can accept treatment while the child or adolescent lives at home; some cannot. Parents are the most important resource for their child, and they must be given the necessary support to fulfill that role. In the past 10 years, a number of innovative models have been developed for providing respite care and in-home intensive services to aid families, especially in times of crisis. When adequate family support is available, many families are able to maintain seriously emotionally disturbed children at home, children who in the past would have been placed in residential or institutional settings (1). In those cases in which parents are not able to aid, tolerate the behavior of, or act in the best interests of their child and the court removes control of a youngster's care from the family, the state becomes the guardian until such time that the parents are again able to perform their role adequately. When the state elects to assume the parental role, it must do so in good faith and with the best service interests of the child and restoration of the family unit as first priorities.

Within the continuum of care, it is necessary to make assurances that the various service components are coordinated, that service needs are assessed, and that missing service gaps are filled. While parents often play this role alone because of the lack of help, the role is best accomplished as a cooperative effort between parents/guardian and a community-based coordinator (or an "identified service resource"). While this is similar to the case manager role in the adult chronic mentally ill service system, it differs in the integral part played by the family and in the frequent use of the juvenile court and school special education teams as aides in case planning. The locus of this coordinator role cannot be pre-determined and should be developed in concert with the major needs of the individual and the availability of such coordinating capacity in the family and/or various community agencies. Without such a primary ser-vice person responsible for coordinating the treatment plan, it is nearly impossible to assure adequate services and proper placement for an in-dividual severely emotionally disturbed child or adolescent.

The services needed by children and adolescents defined as severely emotionally disturbed fall into five major areas. They are mental health care, physical health care, family, education, and environment. The proper care of each individual child relies on a proper balance and integration of these services. None of these five can be viewed in isolation, as each component depends on the others. These needs must be considered in planning for all emotionally disturbed children and adolescents, whether the child is living at home or in a 24-hour care setting.

The service needs of severely emotionally disturbed children and adolescents are differentiated from the needs of those who are less se-verely disturbed by the attention, special quality, and length of time required to provide the services, such as those available in residential settings and in specially designed educational programs. The needs of severely emotionally disturbed children and adolescents are not the same as those for adults. With adults the needs relate to housing, maintenance, and vocational rehabilitation. With youth they relate more to the need for a family or family equivalent and for educational and habilitative services.

Mental health care. This area includes treatment plans geared toward minimizing or alleviating organic and/or purely emotional deficits. Mo-dalities used include psychodynamic, behavioral, group, and family ther-apy as well as psychopharmacologic treatment. These interventions may be performed in any one of a range of settings from outpatient to full-time inpatient or residential care, as dictated by the needs of both patients and their families.

Physical health care. These services are aimed toward maintaining and maximizing physical health, promoting normal growth and devel-opment, and treating any related or concurrent health problems.

Family. The ability of the family or family equivalent to live with a severely emotionally disturbed child or adolescent and act as a corrective agent is crucial in care and treatment planning. In all but a small number of cases, the family is responsible for the day-to-day care and treatment coordination for a large part (if not all) of the course of the disability. For the most part, the greater the family's ability to support the child, the lesser the need for out-of-home care and more extensive interventions.

Education. Mastery of learning is a major task of childhood. Chronic mental illness often makes children and adolescents unavailable for a formal learning experience. Others may have learning or language disabilities. Autistic, psychotic, mentally retarded, or severely behaviorally disordered children each require different types of educational programs, facilities, and staff. There is a special need for carefully coordinating other service efforts with the efforts of the schools, maximizing the programs required under P.L. 94-142, The Education for All Handicapped Children Act.

Environment. Severely emotionally disturbed children and adolescents require special structures to allow them to perform at their optimal level outside of family and educational settings. These include recreational and, when appropriate for adolescents, vocational programs. These programs enhance peer group contact and offer the potential of a full life experience.

Services in these five areas are provided within a continuum of care that includes placement options in both residential and family settings. Some children will move back and forth between the two settings as their individual treatment needs dictate. In making this determination as to the appropriate placement, three basic factors must be evaluated: 1) the capacity of the child or adolescent to function in the family equivalent; 2) the capacity to function in a community-based educational environment; and 3) the capacity to function in the community environment.

The assessment of these capacities requires that a professional team and the family work together to determine the full range of needs and capacities to be dealt with. The professional team must include appropriate input from mental health and physical health care professionals as well as from educational professionals and those from other community agencies. When 24-hour residential care is felt to be most appropriate, such resources must also be included in the planning effort.

The role of the family is of paramount importance in both planning and decision making. Parents are responsible for the welfare of the child or adolescent and must participate in, or at least consent to, a particular treatment plan. The cooperation and participation of the family is a major factor in the long- and short-term success of any treatment plan. The capacity of the family to tolerate and work with the child's problem in support of a treatment plan is a major determinant in the selection of the most promising treatment modalities and resources. At times the ideal treatment plan is a compromise between the family strengths and needs and the patient's psychopathology, needs, and capacities.

The first assessment parameter, *functioning in the family*, requires that the child have a certain level of interpersonal competence. Also, the family or family equivalent must be able to tolerate the troubling symptoms or behavior and support a treatment process. Therefore, the need for structure will be based on both the youngster's level of functioning and the family's ability to establish structure. While the basic concern is that the child receive appropriate treatment for his or her mental illness, it must be remembered that families have a limited ability to protect the child and others from destructive and dangerous behaviors. If family outpatient interventions and/or behavioral management approaches are unsuccessful in mediating the mental illness or in controlling behavior, a more consistent and tightly controlled environment may be necessary. Another concern is that the family or the family equivalent is not made dysfunctional by the youngster's problems. If the family cannot handle the problems that a severely emotionally disturbed child or adolescent introduces, the parents and/or siblings may themselves develop emotional problems or become less functional.

At the same time the child or adolescent is functioning in the family, he or she must also be able to *function in an educational environment*. Learning is a major task of childhood, and every opportunity to learn must be used. If an individual cannot be maintained in a regular classroom, alternatives should be available in the community. These include special classes in regular school settings (which allow for mainstreaming) and, in cases when a child needs further supervision or a more controlled setting, special day programs.

When a child or adolescent is able to live at home and perform in a community school program, he or she must still have the capacity to *function in the community*. As with the family, the community must be able to tolerate the behavior. Difficult-to-control behavior, including delinquent acts, may indicate the need for a more consistent and tightly controlled environment. This environment may be offered in the community by enhancing, through support, the family's ability to control the child or through the use of structure potentially available in the juvenile justice system. Functioning in the community also includes participation in recreational and, where appropriate, vocational activities. This requires the availability of resources that will provide the level of supervision needed by the individual. Of equal concern is the child or adolescent's ability to interact with peers in a nonschool setting. Youngsters with severe emotional problems must have ample opportunity to interact with children their own age, to benefit from positive peer group experiences, and to be protected from negative ones.

When a youngster is not functioning well in a family-based setting, an assessment must be made as to where the problem is: in the family, in the school, and/or in the community. When the treatment needs cannot be met in the family-based setting, community resources should be available for support. If it becomes evident that community-based resources do not meet the family's treatment and support needs, out-of-home placement in the most appropriate treatment setting should be considered.

When a child or adolescent appears unable to function in a family, attempts must be made to alleviate the problems before he or she is placed outside the home. Mental health services for the family or individuals in the family should be made available, including such support services as respite care and homemaker assistance. Partial hospitalization (day treatment or evening or night care) can also be used to help the family and patient live together. When acute hospital care is available along with family crisis intervention, family support services, and therapeutic camps, the need for inappropriate long-term residential care can often be avoided. If these resources are not sufficient within themselves, alternative family situations such as group homes or therapeutic foster homes may allow the child still to receive care in the community, although outside the family. For children who cannot live at home or elsewhere in the community because of the nature of their own or their family's problems, 24-hour care in a hospital or residential treatment center should be available.

If the child cannot function in a community-based educational environment, a decision must be made as to whether the child would be more appropriately placed in a 24-hour care setting even if the child can function in the family. When the child's inability to function in an educational setting is based on educability alone, community-based habilitation programs, workshops, and other sheltered programs should be available as educational alternatives. When such a child is unable to function in these settings, residential care might be needed to meet the child's learning needs.

Lastly, if the individual cannot function in the community, additional support systems should be available. Highly structured and supervised programs can be used to help the youngster spend his or her time outside the family and educational settings in a helpful and productive way. Some adolescents can benefit most from services in less-structured, community-based "alternative" mental health services. Patterned after drop-in centers and runaway houses, such settings can be used by disturbed youths to remove themselves from age-appropriate adolescent and family developmental struggles. This eases one cause of stress in their environments, thus making both them and their parents more amenable to treatment for underlying severe emotional problems. In other cases, interventions in the juvenile justice system, such as probation, may facilitate the treatment process. In cases in which the child cannot function well in the community (usually by exhibiting out-of-control behavior in the community), a residential setting should be considered.

When a full continuum of services is available, the child or adolescent's needs can be continually met in the most appropriate setting. This allows for movement from one level of service to the next as the level of functioning changes. This concept of placement is the most-appropriate, least-restrictive, treatment structure and assures that there is ample opportunity for the youngster in residential care to return to the family and the community when ready and, conversely, when residential care is needed, that it is available.

Twenty-four hour programs in hospitals or residential treatment programs should offer adequate services in all five areas of service concerns: mental health care, physical health care, family, education, and environment. It cannot be assumed that 24-hour supervisory care is adequate therapy within itself. Institutions that provide only a caretaking function are not therapeutic and have no place in the treatment of severely emotionally disturbed children and adolescents. Programs that do not work with the family while the child or adolescent is in care have less chance for a positive outcome.

Mental health care is offered in 24-hour facilities through various treatment modalities. Individual, group, and family therapies along with the use of psychotherapeutic drugs and behavioral and milieu therapies are among the available techniques. Each should be prescribed as part of an overall treatment plan that integrates all the aspects of residential and community-based programs. Environmental concerns are included in residential programs through the milieu process.

A full range of physical health care, including well-child, developmental, and pediatric treatment resources, should be available in all residential settings. While that is self-evident with such medically based problems as anorexia nervosa, the importance of health care is often neglected with other problems, especially in the case of adolescents, whose developmental body changes are often interrelated with their emotional problems.

Family needs are those most often neglected in a 24-hour setting. Because these special placements are often provided on a regional basis, the distance between the home and placement becomes a limiting factor on families' ability to be part of the treatment plan. With those patients who have been placed because of the family's inability to work with them, it may be difficult to engage the family in a constructive way. Yet these families must be reached and worked with. If the family cannot visit the program, community services should be used to work with them. Not to work with the family directly or indirectly is unacceptable. There must be preparation for the youngster's return home.

Educational needs must be met in residential settings. This major life task of children must be individualized to allow optimal learning for each child. A wide range of educational opportunities must be made available to meet the various needs of the individual. If the patient can handle it, a major portion of the day should be devoted to educational activities. Extremely disturbed or retarded children should be offered an individualized, appropriate learning experience.

State-Level Service Delivery

In *Unclaimed Children*, Jane Knitzer (1) analyzed 1980 survey information from mental health departments and their counterparts in all 50 states and the District of Columbia; reviewed relevant professional literature and state studies; analyzed the major federal programs providing funds for disturbed children or affording protection to children and adolescents who need mental health services; and interviewed providers, lawyers, public officials, and child advocates across the country. Her findings at the federal, state, and community levels were both dismal and appalling. She revealed that only a handful of states were even beginning to meet their service responsibilities toward children and adolescents with mental health needs. Furthermore, when states were developing any services for children and adolescents they most frequently focused on

> traditional residential care rather than more cost-effective community-based alternatives. Few mental health departments reflected a policy focus on children and adolescents in their administration, fiscal policies and practices, planning strategies, standard setting, monitoring, training or attempts to protect children's rights and advocate on their behalf. (1, p xi)

Since the publication of Knitzer's report, however, increasing interest has been devoted to the development of a continuum of services for severely emotionally disturbed children and adolescents, both at the federal and state levels. In July 1983, Isaacs (17) conducted a telephone survey of the State Mental Health Representatives for Children and Youth in 47 states and the District of Columbia to determine the current status of mental health service for children and adolescents within the state. For the most part, Isaacs found that States had undertaken, or were in the process of developing, more initiatives for severely emotionally disturbed children than previously found in the March 1981 survey results analyzed by Knitzer. Two years later, many more State Mental Health Authorities seemed to be aware of the major problems and needs of severely emotionally disturbed youth within their States. (18, p 21)

Approximately one-third of the states reported that services for emotionally disturbed children and youth had become a major priority either directly within the state Mental Health Authority or within the legislative or executive branches of state government. Fourteen states, approximately one-third of the states surveyed, indicated that services to emotionally disturbed children and youth were the *top* priority within the Mental Health Authority. An equal number reported that child mental health issues were a major concern to their state legislatures. This interest took the form of specific legislation, resolutions, or the establishment of specific task forces to study the problems. Fourteen states also noted that youth mental health issues were a major concern to the governors of their states. Many governors had established commissions for problem identification, planning, or coordination efforts. Some had also submitted requests for additional funding in their budgets (18, p 21).

It is also important to state that sometimes the judiciary system or the threat of judicial intervention has been the catalyst for the development of more responsive systems of care for severely emotionally disturbed youth. This was the case in North Carolina, South Carolina, Louisiana and Massachusetts. In general, it seems safe to assert that states that have the support and interest of the legislative, executive or judicial branches of government, tend to be more advanced in developing needed services for severely emotionally disturbed children and adolescents. (18, p. 24)

The activities that the states have undertaken on behalf of severely emotionally disturbed children and adolescents fall into two major areas: internal (those activities directed toward modifying or expanding the mental health continuum of care) and external (those activities focused on interagency collaboration including all relevant systems of care). A number of states have moved in both directions simultaneously. Two examples, North Carolina and Georgia, are described below.

Georgia is a unique state to observe because much of the motivation for addressing the needs of severely emotionally disturbed children and youth came through advocacy efforts on the part of traditional voluntary groups.

Involving both the Mental Health Association of Georgia and the Georgia
Junior Leagues who called attention to the problems of children who need
and do not get mental health services, the State responded by setting up
an interagency State level Troubled Children's Committee to plan for and
try to pool resources for seriously disturbed children. . . . (19, p E-7)

The state Mental Health Department, in collaboration with other key
state agencies, funded a number of parallel multisystem interdisciplinary
committees at the community level to serve as placement committees for
"stuck" cases, those for which all other options had been tried and failed.
These committees were composed of local agency directors, who in addition to being able to resolve specific case problems were able to identify
critical administrative barriers to service delivery and to effect policy
change to better serve this population. All of these demonstration committees have reported significant improvement in interagency cooperation and improved service delivery to severely disturbed children.

North Carolina presents another unique situation. This state has
developed an extensive multisystem continuum of care as a result of a
class action lawsuit and subsequent consent decree signed by the governor. This suit (*Willie M. v. Hunt*) was brought on behalf of a class of
seriously disturbed, assaultive, and/or neurologically impaired or multiply handicapped youths. The lawsuit led to a major restructuring of
mental health and related services for that class of children and cata-
pulted North Carolina into a position of leadership in actually implementing systems of care for the specific target group (19).

As a result of the lawsuit, the state must provide habilitation—
including medical services, education, training, and care and treatment
within the least-restrictive, most normal living environment—for Willie
M. and all other members of the class. To do this, North Carolina has
sought to develop a range of specialized services in all its geographical
areas, relying heavily on local assessments of need. To insure that the
individualized habilitation plan is actually carried out, the state has
defined a core role for case managers who, in effect, have been assigned
the responsibility of being case advocates.

The effort to implement the remedies required in *Willie M.* through a series
of court stipulations has not been smooth or easy: there have been administrative and conceptual problems, particularly about the boundaries of the
case manager's role, and the recourse such managers have when service
systems and providers do not respond. But there is also no question that
now, five years after the lawsuit was initially brought, a substantial number
of class members have been served, a range of new services are in place,
and perhaps most significantly, those working with Willie M. clients have

learned that the philosophy undergirding the lawsuit, which holds that no child is untreatable, has proven feasible. Class action litigation is often not the advocacy strategy of choice. It is very costly and frequently, does not show results as rapidly as *Willie M.* has. It can, however, be significant in focusing attention on, and forcing solutions to, an otherwise intractable set of problems that result in legally unacceptable harms to children (19, p E-8)

Federal-Level Service Delivery System Building

As stated before, there have been a number of federal programs that have attempted to develop comprehensive service delivery systems for children and adolescents. Following the Report of the Joint Commission on the Mental Health of Children (2), the Office of Child Development (OCD) was instituted within the Department of Health, Education and Welfare. Growing out of the old Children's Bureau, this office had the mandate to spearhead a nationwide system of advocacy with federal, state, and local components. OCD funded "Offices for Children" in a number of states. Several federal agencies (including OCD, NIMH, the Office of Education, and Social and Rehabilitation Services) developed Child Advocacy programs to meet the recommendations of the commission.

These programs never developed into a system, and by 1984 most of the state offices were disbanded and none of the local projects have survived. However, these programs did help to elucidate the barriers to service delivery that exist.

The major barrier is that the mental health and related services for severely emotionally disturbed children and adolescents are funded through a patchwork system of categorical programs. Each of these programs primarily focuses on one of the components of a comprehensive system. Meanwhile, other components of the system are ignored or, at times, placed in an unrealistic position of being expected to provide "all related services."

The Community Mental Health Centers Program was, from 1963 to 1980, the national program aimed at providing comprehensive mental health services for all persons in need in a local catchment area. Within three years of funding, all new centers were expected to provide (directly or through linkages) the broad comprehensive range of services needed for children and adolescents. Responsibility for linkage with other service systems was not included but was implied in further provisions that require consultation and education services, many of which are provided to schools, courts, and child welfare agencies. Although the requirement of all centers to have children's programs was a major step toward adequate service delivery, it failed to emphasize the integral part played by other service providers. Further, many centers had not developed adequate children's services.

The Education for All Handicapped Children Act, Public Law 94-142, similarly attempts to affect the education system. The act recognizes the broad range of related services, including mental health services, required to assure education programs for all handicapped children, including those with emotional handicaps. Although the act is categorically aimed toward the education of these youngsters, the need for related services is highly visible. A major barrier occurs when the act requires school systems, already fiscally overwhelmed, to assume the burden of assuring that the often extremely expensive services be available. Although the act specifically requires the provision of education and related services at no cost to the parent, it does not specify who *will* bear the costs. In the struggle to provide the funds or to define who is responsible for these services, children in need are often not served or inappropriately served.

The Social Security Act also contains programs that impact on severely emotionally disturbed children and adolescents. Titles IVA and IVB relate to Aid to Dependent Children and child welfare services; Title V relates to maternal and child health programs. Title XIX relates to medical assistance, which includes the Early and Periodic Screening, Diagnosis and Treatment Program, and to reimbursement for inpatient, partial hospitalization, and outpatient services. Title XX offers grants to states that can fund a wide range of welfare-related mental health efforts. These programs are categorical in their focus and as such relate narrowly to special populations as defined by various child welfare mandates. While there is a recognition within all these programs that comprehensiveness is necessary, many barriers to total care are created by meeting that goal through restrictions as to the types of institutions funded under certain programs; for example, hospitalization in some settings (general hospitals) can be funded under Medicaid while comprehensive community mental health centers and group homes cannot. States can further restrict the use of funds in these categories. While the specifics of these acts are not presented here, it is important to understand the great potential in the comprehensive service that has been created only to be severely limited by categorization and in implementation.

Similarly, the Law Enforcement Assistance Administration programming has offered many potential options to youth whose severe emotional disturbance is manifest by a behavior disorder that has been labeled as a status offense or a delinquency. The severe mental illness is not often recognized and attended to in these cases. Further, as is also true with the Runaway Youth Act, the conceptual basis of these programs, which categorize youth on the basis of certain behaviors, limits their usefulness to the care of the most severely emotionally disturbed children and adolescents by embedding them in the juvenile correctional or youth service systems, while neglecting any evident mental illness. An important factor in this barrier is the failure of the mental health system to offer alternatives for these children.

In 1978, the President's Commission on Mental Health recognized these severely emotionally disturbed children and adolescents as an underserved population. When the Mental Health Systems Act, Public Law 96-398, was developed in 1980, an effort was made to encourage the development of more comprehensive services for those populations that were highlighted as underserved by the commission. Under the Mental Health Systems Act the states were required to develop comprehensive care systems for both chronic mentally ill persons and severely emotionally disturbed children and adolescents. A major consideration in this concept was the integration of service delivery, with funding of direct service entities a secondary concern. State plans would have been required to demonstrate how the needs of this population of severely disturbed children and adolescents, including those defined as chronic mentally ill, would be met.

In 1980, the Alcohol, Drug Abuse and Mental Health Block Grant Act replaced the Community Health Center Program, as amended by the Mental Health System Act. Under the Block Grant Act, states are given the responsibility, within broad federal guidelines, to fund community-based mental health services, including those for severely emotionally disturbed children and adolescents. Both the state mental health authorities and Congress recognized that a new approach needed to be taken if the full continuum of care was ever to be developed in communities. In 1984, Congress earmarked $1.5 million to develop a new initiative to improve service delivery for severely emotionally disturbed children and adolescents. The success of the NIMH Community Support Program (CSP) in serving a similar need for chronic mentally ill adults indicated that such a system- and strategy-building approach would also be effective for children. An earlier NIMH program, called the Most in Need (MIN) program, demonstrated that system building on a local level could increase the level, quality, and appropriateness of services received by children.

THE CHILD AND ADOLESCENT SERVICE SYSTEM PROGRAM

From the congressional mandate to develop a new service system initiative for severely emotionally disturbed children and adolescents, NIMH developed the Child and Adolescent Service System Program (CASSP).

CASSP is the natural product of all the definitional, epidemiologic, and service delivery issues presented in this chapter. The major goal for the program is to promote the development of continuua of care for all severely emotionally disturbed children and adolescents in all communities in the country.

In order to meet this goal, the program supports the creation of state-level foci for severely emotionally disturbed children and adolescents (under the auspices of the child mental health authority). All component agencies, public and private, are called upon to become part of a coalition to assure the appropriate provision of services. These agencies include, on the state level: mental health, health, education, welfare, and juvenile justice. Alternative youth services and advocacy groups must also be included as equal partners in this coalition.

From the CSP experience, the concept of advocacy for system development has been incorporated. All parties and agencies interested in meeting the needs of troubled children must learn to work together to 1) identify service gaps and barriers, 2) develop needed service options, and 3) develop mechanisms for overcoming barriers by changing regulations, legislation, and/or established funding patterns.

Once a state has developed comprehensive system building, CASSP promotes the translation of these systems to the community level. As with the child advocacy recommendations of the Joint Commission on the Mental Health of Children 15 years earlier, CASSP is trying to create a system that develops policy at the most effective governmental levels and then utilizes a pyramid system to filter down the policy to local programs and individual children and families. Of course, a major component of this type of system is to develop mechanisms to assure that case-level input is available to the top-level policymakers. Coalitions of service delivery professionals, advocates, and consumers are the necessary participants in this type of process.

CASSP's first task is to ask states to create an office that has a focus on service for severely emotionally disturbed children and adolescents. It asks this office to define the population, perform a needs assessment, develop a plan, and create strategies for the implementation of the plan. All agencies involved with the population should be included at a policy-making level, appropriate for that particular state. States are also asked to develop mechanisms to offer technical assistance to entities (state and local) within their state and in neighboring states.

When this first task has been instituted, although not necessarily completed, states are then asked to demonstrate the same planning and strategy development on a community level. While these local system-building components may be modeled after state-level programs, it is important for community systems to adapt to the unique characteristics of each individual locality. Just as state-level system building is geared to the available strengths and resources within the state agencies and constituencies, communities must build on a similar combination of positive factors.

At the time of the preparation of this chapter, NIMH had just awarded 10 CASSP grants. Some of these proposed expanding relatively sophisticated state systems. Others were from states in which there had previously been no functional child mental health system. While the success of this program has yet to be tested, the concepts hold great promise. A great majority of the states, with or without federal funding, are moving in the directions described in this chapter. Forty-four out of a possible 54 state and territorial entities applied for CASSP grants, even though it was widely known that only 10 could be funded. This desire to develop coherent, appropriate, and comprehensive services for severely emotionally disturbed children and adolescents is at an all-time high. We can now look toward a decade in which major advances in the funding and availability of these services are at hand.

CHILDREN OF THE CHRONIC MENTALLY ILL

Another population of children that requires some special attention is children of chronic mentally ill parents. Children of psychotic and affective-disordered adults have been studied and the risk of these conditions is well accepted. In addition, concern for the results of chronic mental illness on the stability and usefulness of the family has been stated.

Anthony (20) has studied parental psychosis as a psychiatric risk factor in children. He approaches this issue from the perspective of a range of child responses to parental illness. On one hand are the children who are severely affected and on the other hand are those who appear to be "invulnerable" (21). He feels that

> the child's vulnerability is gauged on the degree of involvement with the sick parent and his sickness in terms of identification with the sick parent, knowledge of the illness, undue suggestibility and submissiveness, symptomatic behavior similar to that of the sick parent, and test indications. . . . (20, p 104)

While it is clear that severe emotional illness is a great risk factor, it is also clear that the degree of risk cannot be assumed and must be determined through proper assessment.

Within the range of risk due to parental psychosis, some factors can be attributed to constitutional/genetic factors and some to the developmental effects of growing up with chronic mentally ill parents. The studies of the genetic links within families for schizophrenia (22) and those more recently linking major affective disorders between generations (23) are strong indicators that just being born to a severely emotionally ill parent puts the child constitutionally at risk for equally serious mental illness. Family problems place the child at greater risk for emotional problems. There have not been formal studies of the effects of chronic mental illness as a defined entity on the mental health of the children of this population. While the aforementioned studies relate the risk of various diagnostic entities to problems with children of the affected individuals, none of these studies has taken the degree of parental disability into consideration in trying to understand the risk to the child.

Crystal (24) notes that, in his recent study of homeless women and men, 53 percent of the women had at least one child and 63 percent of these had children under the age of 17. Of these dependent children, half lived with relatives or in other informal living arrangements, while the other half lived in foster care or were institutionalized. This is a large number of affected children just from that portion of the chronic mentally ill population defined as homeless. Similar statistics are not available for the total chronic mentally ill population, but the number of children affected is extremely large, and many of these youngsters require out-of-home placement for long or short periods of time related to the parent's illness.

Studies of the effects of foster care on the emotional status of children have demonstrated significant problems. Murphy (25) describes the "former foster child syndrome." She describes a fear of hurt by society and desire to hurt society back, excessive concern for defenses against these feelings, and a desire for marriage and family without being able to tolerate either. Fanshel and Shinn (26) in their classic study of children in long-term foster care indicate a great number of emotional problems among the placed children. They report that the largest percentage of children going into foster care did so because of the mental illness of a parent. While one cannot automatically assume that most of these parents were chronic mentally ill, a great number of children placed on the basis of mental illness of a parent would most likely come from families of the chronic population. The results of the placement of these children have a profound effect on their emotional well-being and define a major risk factor related to the illness of their parent.

The risk for a child of a chronic mentally ill parent appears to be high; however, more study is necessary to determine the full breadth of the problem. Those who intervene on behalf of the chronic mentally ill must also take into consideration the effects on any children in the family. Case management and treatment planning must provide preventative planning for involved children.

REFERENCES

1. Knitzer J: Unclaimed Children: The Failure of Public Responsibility to Children and Adolescents in Need of Mental Health Services. Washington, DC, Children's Defense Fund, 1982
2. Joint Commission on the Mental Health of Children: Crisis in Child Mental Health: Challenge for the 1970's. New York, Harper and Row, 1970
3. Lourie I, with Fishman M, Hersh S, Platt L, et al: Chronically mentally ill children and adolescents; a special report, in National Plan for the Chronically Mentally Ill. Rockville, MD, National Institute of Mental Health, 1980
4. Kanner L, Rodriguez A, Ashenden B: How far can autistic children go in matters of social adaptation? Journal of Autism and Childhood Schizophrenia 2:9–33, 1972
5. Eggers C: Course and prognosis of childhood schizophrenia. Journal of Autism and Childhood Schizophrenia 8:21–36, 1978
6. American Psychiatric Association: Diagnostic and Statistical Manual of Mental Disorders (Third Edition). Washington, DC, American Psychiatric Association, 1980
7. Gilmore M, Chang C, Coron D: Defining and counting mentally ill children and adolescents. Paper presented at NIMH Workshop on Severely Emotionally Disturbed Children and Adolescents, 1983
8. Toward a National Plan for the Chronically Mentally Ill. Report to the Secretary by the Department of Health and Human Services Steering Committee on the Chronically Mentally Ill (DHHS Publication No. (ADM) 81-1077). Rockville, MD, Department of Health and Human Services, 1981
9. Gould M, Wunsch-Hitzig R, Dohrenwend E: Formulation of hypotheses about the prevalence, treatment and prognostic significance of psychiatric disorders in children in the United States, in Mental Illness in the United States. Edited by Dohrenwend E. New York, Praeger, 1980
10. U.S. Bureau of the Census: General Population Characteristics, Vol. 1. Part 1. United States Summary 1980 Census of Population. Washington, DC, U.S. Government Printing Office, 1983
11. Joint Congressional Commission on Mental Illness and Health: Ac-

tion for Mental Health: Final Report of the Joint Commission on Mental Illness and Health. New York, Wiley, 1961

12. President's Commission on Mental Health: Report of the President's Commission on Mental Health. Washington, DC, U.S. Government Printing Office, 1978

13. Robins L: Psychiatric epidemiology. Arch Gen Psychiatry 35:697–702, 1978

14. Rutter M, Tizard J, Whitmore K: Education, Health, and Behavior: Psychological and Medical Status of Childhood Development. New York, Wiley, 1970

15. Lieberman E: Mental Health: The Public Health Challenge. Washington, DC, American Public Health Association, 1975

16. Silver L: Special mental health needs of children. Options paper prepared for the Select Congressional Panel for the Promotion of Child Health. Washington, DC, 1980

17. Isaacs M: Final Report: A Summary Analysis of Interagency Coordination and Service Integration as Developed Through a Review of the Literature, MIN Projects and State Program Description. Report prepared for the Child and Adolescent Service System Program. Rockville, MD, Alpha Center, National Institute of Mental Health, 1983

18. Isaacs M: Technical Assistance Program for the Child and Adolescent Service System Program, vol. 1. Report prepared for the Child and Adolescent Service System Program. Rockville, MD, National Institute of Mental Health, 1984

19. Knitzer J: Developing systems of care for disturbed children: the role of advocacy. Paper prepared for the Child and Adolescent Service System Program. National Institute of Mental Health, 1984

20. Anthony EJ: A risk-vulnerability intervention model for children of psychotic parents, in The Child in His Family: Children at Psychiatric Risk. Edited by Anthony EJ, Koupernik C. New York, Wiley, 1974

21. Anthony EJ: The syndrome of the psychologically invulnerable child, in The Child in His Family: Children at Psychiatric Risk. Edited by Anthony EJ, Koupernik C. New York, Wiley, 1974

22. Kety S, Rosenthal D, Wender P, et al: Mental illness in the biological and adoptive families of adopted individuals who have become schizophrenic, in Genetic Research in Psychiatry. Edited by Fieve R, Rosenthal D, Brill H. Baltimore, Johns Hopkins University Press, 1975

23. Gershon ES: The genetics of affective disorders, in Psychiatric Update, vol. 2. Edited by Grinspoon L. Washington, DC, American Psychiatric Association Press, 1983

24. Crystal S: Homeless men and homeless women: the gender gap. Urban and Social Change 17:2–6, 1984

25. Murphy L: Long-term foster care and its influence on adjustment to adult life, in The Child in His Family: Children at Psychiatric Risk. Edited by Anthony EJ, Koupernik C. New York, Wiley, 1974
26. Fanshel D, Shinn E: Children in Foster Care. New York, Columbia University Press, 1978

CHAPTER 9

Conclusions and Recommendations

During the first National Conference on the Chronic Mental Patient it was stated that

> there is no more urgent concern than the needs of the chronic mentally ill who suffer from severe, persistent, or recurrent mental illness with residual social and vocational disabilities. As a result of the deinstitutionalization programs of the past decade and the continuing growth of high risk populations that generate chronically ill, the problems associated with the care of these patients constitute a national crisis. (1, p 209)

Unfortunately, today, the problems associated with the care and treatment of the chronic mentally ill continue to constitute an even greater national crisis, due to: 1) the additional social problems related to the increase of the homeless mentally ill population; 2) the increase of a new population called young adult chronic patients; 3) the lack of service for severely emotionally disturbed children and adolescents; 4) the increase of mentally ill persons in correctional facilities; 5) the increase of discrimination against the mentally ill; 6) the lack of significant mental health leadership at the national level; 7) the reduction in training of professionals in community support services, for example, psychiatry, rehabilitation, and psychosocial; 8) the lack of comprehensive community mental health services for the chronic mentally ill; 9) the lack of public funds allocated to serve chronic mentally ill in more least-restrictive environments and to reimburse mental health treatment plans aimed at rehabilitating persons versus reinforcing their weakness and dependence; and 10) the federal government's efforts to limit the number of mentally ill who qualify for federal support under the social security system.

During the past eight years, the mental health field has witnessed new social problems emerging into its service system with the increase and visibility of homeless, young adult chronic patients and severely emotionally disturbed children and adolescents. These populations represent a new challenge and concern for mental health professionals and advocates. The presence of mentally ill, homeless, young adult chronic patients clearly indicates the social and economic problems of the past five years. The increase and visibility of severely emotionally disturbed children and adolescents have come about due to the absence of a national mental health plan for providing and financing comprehensive services.

The homeless persons seem to be visible on every major city street across the nation. The mass media coverage (network news programs, major newspapers, weekly news journals, and so forth) has escalated public concern and controversy among public policy officials. However, the real public debate is "Which government (federal, state, or local) agency is responsible for providing services and what services are needed?" Mental health providers and policymakers cannot avoid this debate. Bassuk et al. stated:

> Just as with deinstitutionalization and the community mental health movement, the issue is less the location of care than the quality of care. All homeless people need humane living conditions, appropriate medical treatment, and extensive psychosocial services, ideally provided in the community and coordinated through case managers. However, without provision of a sophisticated combination of services that accounts for the special characteristics of this population and the relationship of shelters to the mental health system, the plight of the homeless will continue to be desperate. (2, p 1549)

Young adult chronic patients are a new population of mentally ill young adults; they are a transitional generation that is not deinstitutionalized, but uninstitutionalized (3). They are young men and women between the ages of 18 and 35 who have grown to chronologic adulthood with mental and emotional disorders while living in the community. Young chronic patients, for the most part, are severely and persistently impaired in terms of their psychologic and social functioning, but live in the community as opposed to the institution.

Pepper and his colleagues studied a sample of 800 young adults. While the total data from the study are still being analyzed, they have reported the following information from a sample of 152:

48.5 percent of the "chronic" sample are known by their clinicians to have used or abused alcohol and/or other drugs, 7 percent are known to have been involved in a criminal offense involving violence, 11 percent are known to have been involved in a nonviolent criminal offense, 31 percent are still living with their families, only 16 percent have made suicide attempts, 45 percent have rejected specific mental health services recommended by their clinicians, and 51 percent have never been hospitalized. (3, p 39)

With the increase of young adult chronic patients, the mentally ill homeless, and the duration of deinstitutionalization, there has been a large increase of mentally ill persons in correctional facilities, for example, federal, state, county, and city jails and prisons. These populations have become the victims of criminalization of the mentally ill due to the shortage of public housing, public hospital beds, and society's century-old attitude, "out of sight, out of mind." Thus, with the limited community mental health resources and the continual decreasing of state psychiatric beds, some of the mentally ill homeless and young adult chronic patients are being placed into the correctional system instead of the mental health system. If mental health professionals are going to be effective in serving these specialized populations, their professional boundaries and skills must be expanded to include the social service and correctional field.

There are approximately three million seriously disturbed children and adolescents in the United States, with two-thirds of this population not receiving appropriate services. In a recent report sponsored and published by the Children's Defense Fund, Edelman stated that not only were seriously disturbed children and adolescents an ignored population, but federal and state governments had failed to address their needs:

At a time when our national government is seeking to shift more and more obligations onto states and localities, child mental health is a good area in which governors and state legislators can take real leadership. They already have primary responsibility for the fate of these vulnerable children and families. However, with a few exceptions, which we applaud, they have not begun to exercise that responsibility." (4, p vii)

Studies (5, 6) indicate that states continue to provide mostly inpatient services for this population, which are the most restrictive and costly.

PROGRESS AREAS SINCE CONFERENCE

However, the mental health field is appropriately responding to each of the issues listed above through advocacy, research, training, and seeking additional funds. Since the 1978 conference mentioned above, the mental health professional consumers and advocates have made some significant progress in such areas as: 1) the role of the family; 2) the dissemination of psychiatric rehabilitation treatment technology; 3) the development of the National Institute of Mental Health's (NIMH's) Community Support Program (CSP); 4) the establishment of NIMH's Child and Adolescent Service System Program (CASSP); and 5) recent court decisions.

The Involvement of Families

The involvement of families in the mental health system has led to a number of positive changes and has affected the care and treatment of the chronic mentally ill person. Families have also advocated for comprehensive services, the safeguarding of individual rights, and for the increase in federal and state funding. Clinical research (7, 8) has clearly demonstrated that involvement of family members improves the treatment of the chronic mentally ill person. Improving the family members' knowledge and understanding of schizophrenia, as well as their problem-solving and communication skills, improves the family members' ability to support their mentally ill relative.

In 1979, with the formation of the National Alliance for the Mentally Ill, a family support network has been developed in all 50 states. This organization has over 30,000 members. One of its recent presidents, Dr. A. B. Hatfield, stated:

> It has become increasingly clear that the success of the movement toward care of the mentally ill in the community might well depend upon the capacities of families to sustain a large portion of the burden. . . . There is an expectation that the number of families involved will increase for the baby boom population is now reaching the vulnerable age at the same time that the cohort of vulnerable elderly is increasing. All of this is occurring at a time of fiscal restraint and reduction of social programs. (9, p 307)

Due to inadequate services, family members have also become involved in monitoring state hospitals (10). For example, the Western Massachusetts Alliance for Mentally Ill Citizens and the district office of the Massachusetts Department of Mental Health developed a formal system for the families to be trained as monitors in order to monitor the wards of a state psychiatric hospital and give feedback to the administrative staff. As a result of this demonstrative project, Reiter and Plotkin reported:

> It supports the concept that professionals and families working together can strengthen the power of advocacy. The program gives both families and

staff the clout to produce concrete and positive improvements in the delivery of services and the conditions of treatment. It can change the administration of programs and institutions and strengthens the ability of service providers and citizens to accomplish compatible goals. Most importantly, it allows family members to become part of the treatment. (10, p 395)

Dissemination of New Technology

Another area of significant progress has been in the development and dissemination of psychiatric rehabilitation technology and NIMH's Community Support Program. With the funding of the National Institute of Handicapped Research, two research and training centers for the chronic mentally ill were developed, one at Boston University under the direction of Dr. William Anthony and one at the University of California, Los Angeles, under the direction of Dr. Robert Liberman. Both research and training centers have played a key role in developing and disseminating empirically tested rehabilitation treatment technology. NIMH has also funded several training projects for psychiatric rehabilitation practitioners. They first funded Fountain House, which has the largest psychiatric rehabilitation training program in the world (it has, for example, trained staff from 30 different states and 10 different countries). The success of the psychiatric rehabilitation technology has been reported in several scientific and psychologic journals (for example, *Journal of Applied Behavior Analysis, Behaviour Research and Therapy, American Journal of Psychiatry,* and *Psychiatric Research*) and internationally recognized journals (for example, *International Association of Psychosocial Rehabilitation Services* and *World Rehabilitation Association for the Psycho-Socially Disabled*). As a result of this technology, chronic mentally ill persons have a better chance for living more effectively in the community and seeing their independence increase.

Psychiatric rehabilitation technology has also influenced positive changes in the care and treatment of mentally ill persons residing in psychiatric hospitals. Kociemba et al. (11) demonstrated that applying the technology in an inpatient setting increased the patient's chances for surviving in community programs. Bell and Ryan (12) and the Kansas Office of Mental Health and Retardation Services (13) have described a process for implementing a psychiatric rehabilitation model in psychiatric hospitals. The rehabilitation unit accepts transferred patients from other inpatient treatment units and/or directly from community programs. Bell and Ryan (12) reported several immediate advantages: 1) patients develop positive self-esteem and confidence about the future; 2) patients have immediate access to job training and still have the support of the hospital; 3) staff work closer with community providers; and 4) community programs become much more interested in receiving the mentally ill patients because of their experience in a psychiatric rehabilitation unit.

In 1977, NIMH created the CSP. By making available funding contracts to state mental health authorities, NIMH's goal was to help states develop and better coordinate community-based mental health and psychosocial services for the chronic mentally ill. All 50 states, the District of Columbia, and two territories have now received federal CSP funds to stimulate state policies and services for the chronic mentally ill. As a result, CSP has improved state awareness and coordination of public and private resources for the mentally ill by targeting the state-level policymakers.

The CSP model has also brought about an increase of community mental health services for the chronic mentally ill person. It has demonstrated that with appropriate technology, community-based programs can be an alternative to state psychiatric hospitals. The success of the CSP model is contingent on a range of comprehensive services, such as 1) case management; 2) outreach workers; 3) psychosocial components, for example, social clubs, vocational training and placement, social skills training, behavioral family management, medication management, and so forth; 4) 24-hour crisis intervention; 5) housing; and 6) close linkage with state psychiatric facilities and other mental health, medical, and social service providers.

Child and Adolescent Mental Health Services

In 1984, Congress appropriated $1.5 million to develop a new federal and state initiative to improve mental health and human services for severely emotionally disturbed children and adolescents. NIMH created CASSP in response to the mandate of Congress. The major goals of CASSP are: 1) to improve the availability of a continuum of services for severely emotionally disturbed children and adolescents; 2) to develop and/or expand leadership capacity at the state level for child mental health programs; 3) to establish coordination mechanisms with various state departments, providers, and interest groups; and 4) to develop program evaluation capacity. As a result of the success of the first year of funding to 10 states (Alabama, Alaska, Georgia, Hawaii, Kansas, Maine, Mississippi, New Jersey, Ohio, and Wisconsin), the 1985 Congress increased its appropriation for CASSP to $3.9 million, which allowed NIMH to add four new states: Indiana, Nebraska, Pennsylvania, and Vermont.

Major Court Decisions

Since 1978, courts have continued to address legal issues presented by the delivery of mental health services. To a large degree, decisions have attempted to more clearly define the nature of the constitutional liberty interest involved when an individual is involuntarily committed to psychiatric treatment facilities through civil commitment processes.

In cases decided prior to 1978, civil commitment was viewed as a "massive curtailment of liberty" that required careful procedural safeguards similar to those traditionally available to criminal defendants. Examples are *Jackson v. Indiana*, 406 U.S. 715 (1972) (14); *Addington v. Texas*, 441 U.S. 418 (1979) (15); *Lessard v. Schmidt*, 349 F. Supp. 1078 (ED Wis 1972) (16); and *O'Connor v. Donaldson*, 422 U.S. 563 (1975) (17). Although fundamental due process at the time of commitment has remained reasonably settled, courts have not been consistent in their analysis of issues occurring after the patient is admitted. Within the latter category is the right of committed patients to refuse psychotropic medication. In addition to constitutional and statutory liberty interests, there have been important decisions concerning right to treatment and civil liability of professionals for wrongful discharge that affect the chronic mentally ill patient.

Among the most controversial of the liberty issues is the right of committed patients to refuse psychotropic medication. Although based at times on a number of constitutional rights, including the First and Fourteenth Amendments, medication refusals have also been challenged by resort to a liberty argument: the freedom/liberty to avoid unwanted bodily intrusions. Even though the U.S. Supreme Court refused to decide the issue on constitutional grounds [*Mills v. Rogers*, 457 U.S. 291 (1982) (18)], lower federal courts have recognized the right of committed patients to refuse medication in the absence of emergency circumstances. Examples are *Rennie v. Klein*, 462 F. Supp. 1131 (DNJ 1978) (19), and *Rogers v. Okin*, 478 F. Supp. 1342 (D Mass 1979) (20). However, as mentioned earlier, those courts that have addressed the issue on its merits have not decided similar cases in similar ways.

To the extent that many are placing liberty as the first among other social interests, it may still be important for state legislatures to specify exactly what the original commitment decision means. In other words, at the time of ordering commitment did the district judge decide that the patient was dangerous and needed confinement to prevent bodily injury, that the patient was in need of psychiatric treatment, or that the patient was unable to enter into a rational decision-making process with respect to need for treatment? It is because of this uncertainty that some courts have recognized the right of involuntary patients to refuse psychotropic medication. If the patient's ability to make treatment decisions is not presented to the court at the time of commitment, that right may pass unaffected through the commitment process. Therefore, to avoid further confusion and needless additional hearings, legislation designed to clarify the requirements of commitment may be important for the future.

Neither has the U.S. Supreme Court made the right to treatment a constitutional guarantee, as many patient advocates expected prior to 1978. The Court has clearly indicated that committed patients have the right to protection from harm and the minimum training necessary to assist in their own protection. In so doing, the Court has emphasized that the judiciary must give due regard to the exercise of professional judgment in the rendering of psychiatric treatment. More specifically, the Court has held that professional decisions are entitled to a presumption of correctness: *Youngberg v. Romeo*, 457 U.S. 307 (1982) (21).

Of equal importance to the issues of right to privacy, right to treatment, and right to refuse treatment is the potential liability for discharge decisions made by mental health professionals. "Wrongful discharge" and "duty to warn" are the popular names given to such cases. "Patient's liberty" and "wrongful discharge" theories developed simultaneously, one stressing the patient's right to return to the community as soon as possible and the other acknowledging the public's right to be protected from potential dangerous acts. However, the evidentiary tools for determining these issues may be contradictory. For example, in civil commitment cases, patients' attorneys often argue that psychiatrists cannot predict anything, and everything they learn outside of direct observation is hearsay. However, in wrongful discharge cases, plaintiffs' attorneys argue that psychiatrists can predict everything and nothing of psychiatric history is hearsay.

The modern trend is most often attributed to the California ruling in 1976 that required due care for mental health professionals in dealing with the issue of dangerousness, even though it is often referred to as a "duty to warn" case: *Tarasoff v. Regents of the University of California*, 551 P.2d 334 (Cal 1976) (22). The requirement of law for reasonable care in professional practice is well settled and perhaps should have caused little debate when stated in *Tarasoff v. Regents of the University of California*. However, the difficulty of predicting dangerousness and the ethical demands for therapeutic confidentiality have led many to question whether it is reasonable to expect warnings, or any other protective measure, in many of the cases that have been brought before the courts since that time. Thus, courts have again been inconsistent in responding to this issue. Examples are *Lipari v. Sears, Roebuck, and Company*, 497 F. Supp. 185 (D Neb 1980) (23); *Durflinger v. Artiles*, 673 P. 2d 86 (Kan 1983) (24); *Sherrill v. Wilson*, 653 SW 2d 661 (Mo 1983) (25); and *Brady v. Hopper*, 570 F. Supp. 1333 (D 1983) (26).

The impact of wrongful discharge cases on the chronic mentally ill may be to reverse the trend of returning patients to the community as soon as reasonably possible. This may result from fear that an unexpected action by the patient will visit civil liability on the professional responsible for the discharge decision. Of primary concern is identifying which dangerous actions of former patients may result in personal liability. The law does not clearly distinguish between those who are dangerous by choice and those who are dangerous by reason of some mental illness that might have been successfully treated. Nor is future dangerousness easily within the predictive ability of mental health professionals, as has been pointed out by many patient advocates since at least 1972 (27). The dilemma of acknowledging least-restrictive alternatives and wrongful discharge on behalf of the chronic mentally ill continues to be a difficult balancing act for most professionals today.

CONFERENCE II'S RECOMMENDATIONS

Participants in Conference II reviewed the various policy statements and recommendations made in conference I (1, pp 211–220). They felt most of the policies and recommendations were still applicable but additions were needed, such as: 1) full civil rights for the chronic mentally ill; 2) reform of funding mechanisms; 3) utilization of families; 4) emphasis on research in the area of chronic mental illness, including epidemiology, etiology, therapy, and effective service delivery; 5) removal of barriers to assure chronic mentally ill patients access to a full range of medical, psychiatric, rehabilitative, income maintenance, social, employment, and related opportunities and services appropriate to their needs in the least-restrictive setting; 6) each state should produce a plan that guarantees that the needs of the chronic mentally ill patient will be provided for; 7) prohibition of discrimination against chronic mentally ill patients in housing; 8) expansion or establishment of training programs for persons, including family members, in the skills appropriate to the needs of the chronic mentally ill person; and 9) community education should be oriented towards increasing the visibility and status of programs directed to the chronic mental patient, etc.

The following are recommendations to be implemented during the next five years for serving the chronic mental ill population:

The Role of the Federal Government

1. Provide more significant leadership with respect to developing and implementing national policies and funding for mentally ill adults and severely emotionally disturbed children and adolescents.
2. Maintain funding for the mental health block grants, CSP grants, human resource program grants, and CASSP grants and expand technical assistance provided by NIMH in these areas.
3. Develop and implement a comprehensive plan for the mentally ill homeless.
4. Develop a national training center to provide technical assistance and training for state legislatures and state mental health authorities.
5. Provide funding to develop three regional research and training centers on the chronic mentally ill person.
6. Develop a more comprehensive national mental health data base, for example, patient characteristics, cost, and so forth.
7. Provide more research funding in the areas of prevention and psychopharmacology.
8. Provide special student aid to universities that train psychiatrists, psychologists, social workers, and nurses to work with the more specialized and disabled mental health population.
9. Provide training grants to train paraprofessionals on bachelor-degree levels in the mental health field to be case managers.
10. Medicaid waivers and home community-based services need to be more flexible in developing services for the chronic mentally ill person.

The Role of the State Government

11. Create and implement a 10-year financial plan for providing mental health services, for example, the role of state hospitals and community mental health centers, defining the accountability for the care and treatment of the mentally ill, and so forth.
12. Create a "blue ribbon" commission to monitor the implementation of the state's 10-year mental health financial plan.
13. Develop legislation to prevent discrimination against the mentally ill in employment, vocational rehabilitation services, insurance policies, education, housing, and so forth.
14. Develop legislation related to state zoning laws for establishment of residential housing for the mentally ill person.

15. Develop legislation for enacting a bill of rights for the mentally ill person residing in the community.

16. Develop legislation for a protection and advocacy system to ensure the implementation of patient rights and protection of patients from abuse. This could be a part of, for example, the protection and advocacy system created by the Developmental Disability Act.

17. Develop legislation to promote easier, more rapid adjudication procedures regarding mental competency or partial competency, especially when there is an urgent need for rapid appointment of a guardian to act on behalf of the mentally incompetent person.

18. Develop involuntary commitment legislation that emphasizes community support services and that especially authorizes involuntary treatment and care of reluctant mentally ill persons in a variety of outpatient settings.

19. Develop legislation that specifically links institutional and community programs more adequately so that predischarge planning and continuity of care will take place.

Additional Recommendations

20. Service systems for the homeless mentally ill should contain the following services at a minimum: screening and referral, crisis stabilization, comprehensive psychosocial rehabilitation services, transportation, information and evaluation, housing, food, and jobs.

21. Mental health professionals need to recognize the critical importance of involving families and consumers in the care and treatment of the chronic mentally ill person and in determining public policy at both the federal and state levels, as well as using families and consumers as external monitors of state hospitals and community mental health center programs.

22. More research is needed to explore prevention and cures of mental illness; for example, this research effort needs to be developed and funded through private funds from citizen contributions and private foundations.

23. The American Psychiatric Association should take the lead in bringing the various mental health disciplines together to discuss training professionals to work with the chronic mentally ill.

24. The definition of a chronic mentally ill person should include a more functional component and be more specific than that utilized in the current *Diagnostic and Statistical Manual of Mental Disorders (Third Edition)* (28) methodology; for example, the definition needs to be tied to diagnostic-related groups.

25. The housing policy as developed by the National Association of State Mental Health Program Directors (see Appendix C) should be implemented.
26. The homeless policy as developed by the National Association of State Mental Health Program Directors (see Appendix C) should be implemented.
27. Services for severely emotionally disturbed children and adolescents need to be comprehensive enough to provide for a wide range of long-term severe disabilities. The components of such a system should include family and community-based resources as well as acute, intermediate, and long-term 24-hour programs.

REFERENCES

1. Talbott JA (ed): The Chronic Mental Patient: Problems, Solutions, and Recommendations for a Public Policy. Washington, DC, The American Psychiatric Association, 1978
2. Bassuk EL, Rubin L, Lauriat A: Is homelessness a mental health problem? Am J Psychiatry 141:1546–1550, 1984
3. Pepper B, Ryglewicz H (eds): Advances in treating the young chronic patient. New Directions for Mental Health Services, no. 21. San Francisco, Jossey-Bass, 1984
4. Edelman MW: Preface, in Unclaimed Children: The Failure of Public Responsibility to Children and Adolescents in Need of Mental Health Services. By Jane Knitzer. Washington, DC, Children's Defense Fund, 1982
5. President's Commission on Mental Health: Task Panel Reports, vol. II. Washington, DC, U.S. Government Printing Office, 1978
6. National Institute of Mental Health: Eighth Annual Report on Child and Youth Activities. Washington, DC, U.S. Government Printing Office, 7 October 1980–30 September 1984 (mimeographed)
7. Falloon IRH, McGill C, Boyd J: Behavioral Family Management. Baltimore, Johns Hopkins University Press, 1984
8. Vaughn CE, Leff JP: The influence of family and social factors on the course of psychiatric illness. Br J Psychiatry 129:125–137, 1976
9. Hatfield AB: The family, in The Chronic Mental Patient: Five Years Later. Edited by Talbott JA. Orlando, FL, Grune and Stratton, 1984, p 395
10. Reiter M, Plotkin A: Family members as monitors in a state mental hospital. Hosp Community Psychiatry. 36:393–395, 1985
11. Kociemba AB, Cotter PG, Frank MA: Predictors of community tenure of discharged state hospital patients. Am J Psychiatry 136:1556–1561, 1979

12. Bell MD, Ryan ER: Integrating psychosocial rehabilitation into the hospital psychiatric services. Hosp Community Psychiatry 35:1017–1023, 1984
13. Kansas Office of Mental Health and Mental Retardation: Program/Budget document, 1984
14. *Jackson v. Indiana.* 406 U.S. 715 (1972)
15. *Addington v. Texas.* 441 U.S. 418 (1979)
16. *Lessard v. Schmidt.* 349 F. Supp. 1078 (ED Wis 1972)
17. *O'Connor v. Donaldson.* 422 U.S. 563 (1975)
18. *Mills v. Rogers.* 457 U.S. 291 (1982)
19. *Rennie v. Klein.* 462 F. Supp. 1131 (D NJ 1978)
20. *Rogers v. Okin.* 478 F. Supp. 1342 (D Mass 1979)
21. *Youngberg v. Romeo.* 457 U.S. 307 (1982)
22. *Tarasoff v. Regents of the University of California.* 551 P.2d 334 (Cal 1976)
23. *Lipari v. Sears, Roebuck and Company.* 497 F. Supp. 185 (D Neb 1980)
24. *Durflinger v. Artilles.* 673 P. 2d 86 (Kan 1983)
25. *Sherrill v. Wilson,* 653 SW 2d 661 (MO 1983)
26. *Brady v. Hopper.* 570 F. Supp. 1333 (D 1983)
27. Ennis BJ: Prisoners of Psychiatry. New York, Harcourt, Brace, and Jovanovich, 1972
28. American Psychiatric Association: Diagnostic and Statistical Manual of Mental Disorders (Third Edition). Washington, DC, American Psychiatric Association, 1980.

Appendix A

AGENDA
NATIONAL CONFERENCE ON THE
CHRONIC MENTAL PATIENT II
August 12–14, 1984
Kansas City International Airport Hilton Hotel

Please Note: This is to be a working conference for which position papers have been prepared ahead of time on six topics, and at which participants will be expected to discuss in small group meetings three of the six topics. Participants will receive advance copies of the three papers their group will be discussing. The scheduled topics are:

Topic I —Who are the chronic mentally ill? What changes have we seen in the last 10 years? What trends do we see?—Howard Goldman, M.D., Ph.D./Ronald W. Manderscheid, Ph.D., National Institute of Mental Health (NIMH).

Topic II —Who are the homeless? What are their needs? What trends do we see?—Leona Bachrach, Ph.D., Research Professor of Psychiatry, University of Maryland School of Medicine.

Topic III—What are the innovative treatment techniques in the Community Support Program model that work to meet the needs of clients with chronic mental illness?—Robert P. Liberman, M.D., Professor of Psychiatry, UCLA School of Medicine.

Topic IV—What are the obstacles to implementing programs for the chronic mentally ill? What are the financial and control issues in providing services for the chronic mentally ill (state versus federal)? What are the legal issues associated with providing services for the chronic mentally ill? What are the problems associated with societal stereotypes of persons with chronic mental illness?—Joseph Bevilacqua, Ph.D., Commissioner of Mental Health and Retardation, commonwealth of Virginia.

Topic V —What is the role of nonprofessionals (for example, ex-patients and families) in providing care and support for the chronic mentally ill client?—Shirley Starr, Co-Founder and Past President, National Alliance for the Mentally Ill.

Topic VI—Who are the children with chronic mental illness, where are they, what are their needs and their rights?—Ira S. Lourie, M.D., NIMH.

Sunday, August 12, 1984

Late —Participants arrive at Kansas City International Airport.
afternoon Take courtesy transportation to International Airport Hilton Hotel.

6:00 p.m. —Social hour (room to be designated by hotel).

7:00 —Dinner. Keynote Address—John A. Talbott, M.D., President, American Psychiatric Association (APA); Professor of Psychiatry, Cornell University Medical College; original Chair, APA Committee on the Chronically Mentally Ill. "The Chronic Mental Patient: Five Years Later."

Monday, August 13

8:00 a.m. —Continental breakfast (room to be designated by hotel).

8:30 —Plenary meeting of all conference participants. Introduction and Overview—W. Walter Menninger, M.D.

9:00 to —Review of conference papers by working committees.
11:30
Session I
(The conference participants will be assigned to one of six committees, each composed of roughly 10 persons. Each committee will have three working sessions of two and a half hours, which a working paper author and a recorder/reporter will attend. Over the course of this day, each committee will discuss three of the six working papers and offer observations, suggestions, and recommendations.
During this first session, Committee A will discuss Topic I; Committee B, Topic II; Committee C, Topic III; Committee D, Topic IV; Committee E, Topic V; and Committee F, Topic VI.

12:00 —Luncheon
Noon —Remarks by Marcia Lovejoy, Director, Project Overcome, Minneapolis, Minnesota. "Recovery from Schizophrenia: A Personal Odyssey" (room to be designated by hotel).

2:00 to —*Session II*
4:30 p.m. Committee review and discussion of prepared papers.
Committee A will discuss Topic II; Committee B, Topic III; Committee C, Topic IV; Committee D, Topic V, Committee E, Topic VI; and Committee F, Topic I.

6:00 p.m.—Dinner for entire group (no program) (room to be designated by hotel).

7:00 to   —*Session III*
9:30 p.m.   Committee review and discussion of prepared papers.
     Committee A will discuss Topic III; Committee B, Topic IV; Committee C, Topic V; Committee D, Topic VI; Committee E, Topic I; and Committee F, Topic II.

Tuesday, August 14

8:00 a.m.—Continental breakfast (room to be designated by hotel).

8:30 to   —Plenary session for all participants.
12:00
noon

8:30   —General remarks and summary statement.

8:40   —Report on Topic I—Ronald Manderscheid/David Cutler.

9:10   —Report on Topic II—Leona Bachrach/Steve Lyrene.

9:40   —Report on Topic III—Robert Liberman/Arthur Meyerson.

10:10   —Break.

10:30   —Report on Topic IV—Joseph Bevilacqua/Neal Brown.

11:00   —Report on Topic V—Shirley Starr/Don Horner.

11:30   —Report on Topic VI—Ira Lourie/Blanca Badillo de Loubriel.

12:00   —Lunch (room to be designated by hotel).
Noon to
1:00 p.m.

1:30   —Summation and recommendations—Walt Menninger/Gerald Hannah.

3:00 p.m.—Adjourn.

Participants in the Conference on the
Chronic Mental Patient II

Ahr, Paul R., Ph.D., M.P.A.
Director
Department of Mental Health
Jefferson City, MO

Bachrach, Leona, Ph.D.
Associate Professor of Psychiatry
University of Maryland School of
     Medicine
Rockville, MD

Bevilacqua, Joseph, Ph.D.
Commissioner
Department of Mental Health and
  Mental Retardation
Richmond, VA

Bowker, Joan P., Ph.D.
Council on Social Work Education
New York, NY

Brada, Donald R., M.D.
Medical Director
Horizons Mental Health Center
Hutchinson, KS

Brown, Neal, M.P.A.
Community Support and
  Rehabilitation Branch
National Institute of Mental Health
Rockville, MD

Budd, Sue
Project Acceptance
Lawrence, KS

Callahan, James J., Ph.D.
Commissioner
Department of Mental Health
Boston, MA

Cassidy, Kathleen
Director
Office of Program Development
Division of Mental Health and
  Hospitals
Trenton, NJ

Clark, Betsy
Larned State Hospital
Larned, KS

Clemmons, J.R., M.D.
Deputy Commissioner
Department of Mental Health/
  Mental Retardation
Austin, TX

Concannan, Kevin
Commissioner
Department of Mental Health and
  Mental Retardation
Augusta, ME

Cutler, David, M.D.
Associate Professor of Psychiatry
Oregon Health Sciences University
Portland, OR

Daniels, LaVonne
Director
Department of Public Institutions
Community Support Program
Lincoln, NE

Danley, Karen, Ph.D.
Boston Center for Research and
  Training
Boston, MA

de Loubriel, Blanca Badillo, M.D.
Child Fellow, University of
  New Mexico
Albuquerque, NM

Doebler, George, Th.D.
Executive Director
Mental Health Clergy
Knoxville, TN

Donohue, Mary
The Menninger Foundation
Topeka, KS

Dyer, Barbara
Mental Health and Retardation
  Services
Topeka, KS

Ferguson, Christine
Manchester, MO

Ferron, Fred, M.D.
Anoka State Hospital
Anoka, MN

Folsom, James, M.D.
Colmery-O'Neil VA Medical Center
Topeka, KS

Gardine, Roberta
CSP Director
Division of Comprehensive
  Psychiatric Services
Department of Mental Health
Jefferson City, MO

Gardner, Jerome R.
Horizon House
Philadelphia, PA

Goodrick, David, Ph.D.
Director
Mental Health Office
Department of Mental Health and
  Social Services
Madison, WI

Griffith, Harriett
President
Kansas Mental Health Association
Wichita, KS

Hannah, Gerald T., Ph.D.
Commissioner
Kansas State Office of Mental
  Health and Retardation Services
Topeka, KS

Harder, Robert C.
Secretary
Social and Rehabilitation Services
Topeka, KS

Horner, R. Don, Ph.D.
Director
Clinical Programs
Mental Health and Retardation
  Services
Topeka, KS

Kennedy, Larry, M.D.
Kansas Mental Health Association
Topeka, KS

Larson, Jan, M.S.W.
The Menninger Foundation
Topeka, KS

Lee, Gwendolyn, M.D.
Medical Director
Osawatomie State Hospital
Osawatomie, KS

Levine, Irene Shifren, Ph.D.
Coordinator
Program for the Homeless
  Mentally Ill
National Institute of Mental Health
Rockville, MD

Liberman, Robert P., MD
Professor
University of California, Los
  Angeles, School of Medicine
Director, Mental Health Clinical
  Research Center
Los Angeles, CA

Lourie, Ira S., M.D.
Deputy Chief
Office of State and Community
  Liaison
National Institute of Mental Health
Rockville, MD

Lovejoy, Marcia
Project Overcome
Minneapolis, MN

Lyrene, Steve, M.D.
Karl Menninger School of
  Psychiatry
Topeka, KS

Manderscheid, Ronald W., Ph.D.
Chief
Survey and Systems Research
  Branch
National Institute of Mental Health
Rockville, MD

McGowan, Sherry
Administrator
Community Support Program
Mental Health and Retardation
  Services
Topeka, KS

McNaught, Thomas, M.D.
Topeka State Hospital
Topeka, KS

Menninger, Karl, II
Department of Mental Health
Jefferson City, MO

Menninger, Walt, M.D.
Executive Vice President and Chief
  of Staff
The Menninger Foundation
Topeka, KS

Metzger, Arlene
President
Families for Mental Health
Topeka, KS

Meyerson, Arthur, M.D.
Mt. Saini Hospital
New York, NY

Miller, David
Project Officer
Community Support and
   Rehabilitation Branch
National Institute of Mental Health
Rockville, MD

Nikkel, Larry W.
Executive Director
Prairie View Mental Health Center
Newton, KS

Ogren, Kenneth
The Menninger Foundation
Topeka, KS

Paul, Gordon L., Ph.D.
Mental Health Services
Houston, TX

Platman, Stanley R., M.D., M.A.
Assistant Secretary, Mental Health
   and Retardation/Developmental
   Disability
Baltimore, MD

Posternack, Melwyn L., M.D.
Medical Director
Mental Health Office
Philadelphia, PA

Prevost, James A., M.D.
Department of Mental Health and
   Mental Retardation
Richmond, VA

Quaison, Nora, M.D.
Medical Director
Rainbow Mental Health Facility
Kansas City, KS

Rein, Bill, J.D.
Legal Counsel
Mental Health and Retardation
   Services
Topeka, KS

Roth, Dee
Chief
Program Evaluation and Research
Department of Mental Health
Columbus, OH

Rubenstein, Leonard
Director
Mental Health Law Project
Washington, DC

Ruttinger, Eunice
Administrator
Community Mental Health
   Programs
Mental Health and Retardation
   Services
Topeka, KS

Schmidt, James
President
Fountain House, Inc.
New York, NY

Sheehan, Ann
National Alliance for the
   Mentally Ill
St. Louis, MO

Snyder, Howard
Past President
Families for Mental Health
Prairie Village, KS

Snyder, Lou
Families for Mental Health
Prairie Village, KS

Starr, Shirley
Co-Founder and Past President
National Alliance for the
   Mentally Ill
Evanston, IL

Talbott, John, M.D.
Professor of Psychiatry
Cornell University Medical Center
New York, NY

Templeman, Harold
Deputy Director
Division of Mental Health, Mental
   Retardation and Developmental
   Disabilities
Department of Social Services
Des Moines, IA

Uliss, Isaiah
Massachusetts Advisory Council on
   Mental Health/Mental
   Retardation
Boston, MA

Wiebe, David, M.S.
Executive Director
Shawnee Community Mental
   Health Center
Topeka, KS

Wilder, Jack F., M.D.
Greenwich, CT

Willsie, Clinton D.
Director
Sedgwick County Department of
   Mental Health
Wichita, KS

Young, Dwight
Executive Director
The Center for Counseling and
   Consultation
Great Bend, KS

Appendix B

Working Papers from the National Conference on the Chronic Mental Patient II

Editors' note: The conference format included small group discussion of six position papers, each on a different topic, with a recorder assigned to accompany each author and summarize the discussion. For two papers, the recorders concluded that the discussion simply reinforced the major observations and conclusions of the authors; thus no additional working paper was drafted for these topics. These two papers were "What are the innovative treatment techniques in the Community Support Program model that work to meet the needs of clients with chronic mental illness?" (Topic III) and "Who are the children with chronic mental illness, where are they, and what are their needs and their rights?" (Topic VI).

Summary Report of Topic I

Epidemiology of Chronic Mental Disorder: Reactions and Recommendations

David L. Cutler, M.D., Recorder, and
Ronald W. Manderscheid, Ph.D.

This conference was designed to go beyond the initial national conference. Indeed, the addition of patients and patient advocates as presenters and participants added perspectives not previously well identified. The results of the discussion of this topic by three small groups reflect the complex problem of trying to fit a specific definition of chronic mental illness into a pluralistic society with a wide variety of points of view. The groups and the individuals within them did not necessarily agree, either on definitions or recommendations. We present these ideas, nonetheless, in the hope that they may add perspective for planners, mental health administrators, legislators, family members, and patients who are concerned with the future development of adequate public programs for chronic mentally ill persons, both in and out of institutions.

Reviewing several key points of the position paper, Manderscheid noted the difficulty in defining and counting the chronic mentally ill. Different agencies frequently have a different method of defining these patients; for example, the National Institute of Mental Health (NIMH) Community Support Program defines chronic mental illness one way, and entitlement programs such as Supplemental Security Income, Social Security Disability Insurance, and state and mental health agencies define it in other ways. All do use one or more of the three basic elements: diagnosis, disability, and duration.

NIMH estimates some three million people have a *diagnosis* that falls into a category that might be considered chronic mental illness. Relevant diagnoses include schizophrenia, major affective disorders, paranoid disorders, other psychotic disorders, and certain organic mental disorders. Currently, of those three million who have a relevant diagnosis, an estimated 2.4 million also have some sort of functional *disability* that prevents them from being able to work and may also cause other problems in basic areas of living such as self-care, social interaction, and learning ability. Finally, approximately 1.7 million of this population have been disabled for a significant *duration*, a period of time sufficient to qualify for state services. Typically, duration is defined in terms of length of hospitalization; for example, the NIMH Community Support Program defines its target population as persons who have had a single episode of psychiatric hospitalization in the last five years of at least 6 months' duration or two or more hospitalizations in a 12-month period. In the state of Oregon, chronic mentally ill persons are defined by having a diagnosis and also some impaired role functioning in social situations, daily living skills, or social acceptability; however, in order to receive intensive case management, a person also needs to be a high bed-day utilizer at the state hospital (30 bed-days/year) (Bigelow and Gareau 1983).

Clearly, many chronic mentally ill people have not been served by the system in order to receive a diagnosis, nor have they been admitted to hospitals. For example, jails, voucher hotels, and shelters for the homeless are common places where one may find patients who are not called patients. According to the U.S. Department of Housing and Urban Development, about one-third of the so-called homeless in America are chronic mentally ill. This averages roughly 185,000 people on any given day. The National Coalition for the Homeless estimates 2.2 million homeless persons per year, of which roughly half are chronic mentally ill. Since the states and the federal government entitlement programs have different ways of defining the chronic patients and also have different priorities as to how to deal with them, the result is significant discontinuity of service and financial support for persons with certain kinds of problems. Others, because of their inability or unwillingness to contact the formal mental health system, are never diagnosed and admitted to care. Should these people have services, or should they be allowed to avoid the system? Is it in their best interest to allow them no treatment?

Are there better ways to define the chronic mentally ill? Dr. Manderscheid observed that planners, funders, and providers have largely been concerned only with person variables. Setting, provider, and treatment variables could also play a role in determining who is included in the population. For example, the prevailing definitional elements of diagnosis, disability, and duration reflect two person variables and one setting variable (that is, length of inpatient stay). To date, no one has ever utilized provider variables or treatment variables to define the population. Further, there are problems with the definitional elements generally used. For instance, should not some nonpsychotic disorders of long duration be included in the category, as well as all lasting organic mental disorders? With regard to disability and levels of functioning, there may be wide differences among persons' capacity for personal care. Some may have difficulty in basic care (that is, taking care of dress, food, clothing, and personal hygiene), while others are simply limited in the capacity to sustain complex levels of personal care (going shopping, buying food, going to the bank, using public transportation, writing, and so forth). Similarly, there are different levels of social functioning, one involving activities that can be done alone (watching television, playing solitaire) and others that require some interaction (sports, bridge).

Given these underlying definitional problems, the conference discussion groups focused on a number of topics: 1) stigma, 2) barriers to service, 3) service system comprehensiveness, 4) definitions and funding issues, and 5) training and education of professionals.

STIGMA

Many discussants felt that those responsible have not done a good job of defining the chronic mentally ill, since on the one hand we seem to exclude large numbers of people in need of help, and on the other hand those who are included often receive more stigma than treatment. Sue Budd, of Project Acceptance, pointed out, "What do we need a definition for? I have had six diagnoses in my life. Is it really definable? I believe it is a problem that people are forced into a system and then iatrogenically trapped in it. I am concerned about entrapment of the mentally ill in ineffective, overly restrictive, outmoded settings." The issue of entrapment goes beyond that of depriving a person of his rights and placing him in a hospital. It is also a situation where a person is forced to deal with a stigmatizing public service system that only responds if a person is deemed "chronic" and thus forces a patient into proving chronicity. The counterpoint to this is the chronic patients who somehow avoid being counted. The latter includes those who live with families and do not receive mental health services. Mrs. Howard Snyder, of Families for Mental Health, pointed out "My son is a chronic mental patient, and although the Community Support Program is great, he can't get into the hospital when he needs it. He is one of those young and educated chronic patients, who continues to get sicker every day." Dee Roth, of the Ohio Department of Mental Health, pointed out that advocates need to be able to tell their legislatures who the chronic patients really are, as providers are no longer effective or well received due to their being perceived as "special interest groups" within the system. Unresolved by the discussants was how to better define the chronic mentally ill so as to encourage legislators to fund programs without causing further stigma.

BARRIERS TO SERVICE

A significant problem is presented by those chronic mental patients who are "institutionalized" in their own homes. A common denominator with these patients is their enormous dependency, combined with our society's aversion to and denial of the existence of dependent people. If we lived in a culture that did not have trouble tolerating dependency, we would not have to attach specific criteria to define the chronic patient, and anyone who did not function very well would be eligible for some kind of government subsidy, dole, or entitlement program. In such a case, the issue of definition of the chronic patient would be a moot point. Since we do not live in such a society, we must go to some trouble to define adequately which persons should get services. The consensus was clear that the long-term care of the chronic mentally ill should not simply be left to their families. These families can be sorely taxed by the ill dependent and need periodic respite or vacations from caring for their ill family member. Parents caring for a chronic mentally ill child are also concerned that when they die no one will be left to care for their child. Complicating the problem is the fact that many children living with their parents are not defined as chronic mentally ill since their personal (family) support system is somehow able to manage them. These families see the state hospital as a major source of asylum for their ill dependent, but unless he/she is "dangerous," he/she may not be eligible for hospital admission.

In addition to patients who have become institutionalized in their homes, another population consists of those chronic mentally ill who are now stabilized in mental health centers, requiring either a small amount of therapy and/or additional psychotropic medication without much else in the way of support. These people are diagnostically chronic patients, but they do not fit the criteria for functional disability or duration of stay in hospitals. Since more funding emphasis is now being focused on chronic and severely mentally ill persons who fit the criteria, those persons who do not fit but who are already in treatment run the risk of losing services that are helping them to survive, thereby becoming more chronically mentally ill, going through the revolving door of hospitals, and developing disabilities they do not now have.

SERVICE SYSTEM COMPREHENSIVENESS

Problems of stigma and dependency raise the question: what should the ideal service system be like? How can we get resources to fund such a system? Is cost effectiveness the only watchword, or should we consider treatment system effectiveness? With regard to medical or psychological rehabilitation and support systems, how should these systems be structured? Should they include patient-run social clubs? Should they include day programs operated by community mental health centers? Should patients be involved in church socialization groups, recreation groups, psychosocial rehabilitation programs, and so forth? Discussants felt if a spectrum of services were available, all chronic patients would take advantage of them without having to be defined as chronic mentally ill. This might include many patients who are not definable by the system because they are being maintained and supported by their own families and are not as dependent on the community treatment services.

In fact, mental health delivery systems are highly fragmented and devoid of major elements that are necessary to provide adequate care in the community. There is not enough system "glue" despite the development of case management. There are an insufficient number of physicians, some of whom are not adequately trained to be active both in providing medications and in consultative and programmatic contact with elements of the support system. Further, there need to be better community living arrangements, better working environments, and better social environments for chronic patients. The lack of all these elements makes it difficult to determine what the needs of the patient really are, since the patients cannot be observed and evaluated in environments appropriate for them.

DEFINITION AND FUNDING ISSUES

Dr. James Prevost observed that we need to find a way to settle on definitions and not argue too much about problems with defining. With the advent of diagnostic related groups (DRGs), persons will simply not be eligible for service without a diagnosis. However, it is not easy to tie a psychiatric diagnosis to funding in a realistic manner. Many discussants felt that the diagnosis should include a functional component somewhat more specific than that utilized in the current psychiatric diagnostic manual (American Psychiatric Association 1980) methodology. In addition, access to services should be related to the presence or absence of supportive network elements; for example, schizophrenia with no friends, relatives, family, or other supports is different and costs more in resources than schizophrenia with friends, relatives, families, a job, and recreation. There is no question that the lack of a support group increases the length of hospitalization.

TRAINING AND EDUCATION OF PROFESSIONALS

A major problem with delivering services to the chronic mentally ill is the lack of incentive for traditional mental health worker training programs to focus on the problems of these patients. In past years, NIMH provided grants to schools of social work, psychology, psychiatric nursing, and psychiatry to upgrade training in community support systems focused on the chronic patient. These grants have disappeared; and as the years go by, the impact of that lost funding will become more and more apparent. With specific reference to physicians, an increasing emphasis in training on biologic-medical model approaches prompts new psychiatrists to feel uncomfortable dealing with social and interpersonal issues. Yet the critical role of the psychiatrist on the treatment team makes it imperative that he or she understand enough about social psychiatry to recognize the impact that social support systems have on the functioning of chronic mentally ill persons. To care effectively for these patients, physicians need training in social psychiatry (Cutler et al. 1981). Meanwhile, who will the case managers of the next generation be? Will it be possible to use existing private-sector family practitioners to act as case managers for those chronic patients who are no longer disabled and who could be mainstreamed into the general medical population? In the British system, the general practitioner is the ultimate case manager for all patients except the more complicated psychiatric patients. If we are to move in this direction, we will need to educate general practitioners about the long-term care of the chronic mentally ill.

CONCLUSIONS AND RECOMMENDATIONS

1. We need better definitions, probably tied to DRGs.
2. We need to recognize that patient needs have to be evaluated in terms of realistic goals and timetables.

3. We need a method of determining which mentally ill persons are going to require indefinite care and how we identify them.
4. Since stigma is a major problem and will continue to be so, we need to develop ways to get the community to accept chronic mental illness and to allow chronic patients to be involved in everyday activities.
5. We need to define more adequately what we mean by level of functioning and build that into the environments that we have available for chronic patients.
6. We need to find a way to measure environments better.
7. We need to consider an ideal system such as the Balanced Service System, which is now being used by the Joint Commission on Accreditation of Hospitals to evaluate community mental health programs, as a standard for programs for the chronic mentally ill.
8. We need to develop pragmatic operational research in these areas. The Balanced Service System approach might be one way to frame this research.

To achieve some of these ends, we suggest the following *action* steps:

1. Community education.
2. Developing stronger partnerships between advocates and providers.
3. Implementing a better level of organization at the legislative lobbying level.
4. Studies of natural environment programs that provide cost savings in order to differentiate more clearly the costs of different levels of care such as residential programs, day programs, socialization, and psychosocial rehabilitation.
5. Finding ways to work within the private sector such as a state demonstration grant to provide a prospective payment system for health maintenance organizations.
6. Getting involved with the definition of DRGs, so that they would be able to support long-term care for those patients who need it.
7. Provide advocacy for patients so that they can qualify for the various entitlement programs necessary in order for them to survive in the community (for example, should states continue to try to get Medicare waivers to use for day care and other nonhospital treatment?).
8. Advocate for better outcome measures, both in terms of the effects of environmental factors and rehabilitation on role performance.

With the current climate in the country, these action steps will be difficult to achieve. Nonetheless, there has never been as much opportunity for unity among patients, family members, and providers. We hope that this new alliance can maintain itself and continue to strive towards these mutually beneficial goals.

REFERENCES

American Psychiatric Association: Diagnostic and Statistical Manual of Mental Disorders (Third Edition). Washington, DC, American Psychiatric Association, 1980

Bigelow D, Gareau M: Implementation and effectiveness of the Dammasch bed reduction project. Oregon Mental Health Division, Program Analysis Section, May 1983

Cutler DL, Bloom JD, Shore JH: Training psychiatrists to work with community support systems for chronically mentally ill persons. Psychiatry 138:98–101, 1981

Summary Report of Topic II

Who are the homeless? What are their needs? What trends do we see?

Steve Lyrene, M.D., Recorder

In looking at the problems of the homeless mentally ill, one soon realizes that these issues are complex, our knowledge is limited, and the viewpoints about these problems and possible approaches to them are quite varied. In three sessions led by Dr. Leona Bachrach on August 13, 1984, committees sought to examine these issues, to share facts and experiences, and to explore possible ways to address the problems.

Each of these three sessions primarily addressed different aspects of the problems of the homeless mentally ill in a way which naturally developed the topic. The morning session focused on issues of definition, description, and a listing of the needs of the homeless mentally ill. The afternoon session focused on barriers that prevent the chronic mentally ill, especially the homeless, from utilizing mental health care and its resources. The evening session focused on policy issues affecting this population. The discussions led to a clearer conceptualization of the problems, and a general framework from which to approach the problems was proposed. The following gives a brief overview of the discussions in the three sessions:

Defining the term "homeless chronic mentally ill" is difficult, for there is a precise definition for neither "homeless" nor "chronic mentally ill." Does homeless mean without shelter? Or without affiliation? Or both? "Chronic mentally ill" formerly referred to a long history of institutionalization. But in this era of deinstitutionalization, that is no longer an effective definition. For purposes of discussion, however, the homeless chronic mentally ill can be looked at as the undomiciled chronic mentally ill.

In approaching the study of the homeless chronic mentally ill, it is important to know whether this group is being conceptualized as a subgroup of the mentally ill (the homeless mentally ill) or as a subgroup of the homeless (the mentally ill homeless). One's orientation affects research approaches and treatment planning with this group.

Where did the homeless chronic mentally ill come from? A number of factors have led to an increase in their numbers. Because of the baby boom, greater numbers of people are now at an age of increased risk for severe mental illness. In the past they would have been hospitalized. Now they are hospitalized only a short time or not at all, and they are highly visible. They have more access to street drugs and more mobility, which makes them more visible; and the lack of the counterculture of the sixties takes away their cover and also makes them more visible. Thus, now there are more homeless people than ever, a greater percentage of these people are the homeless mentally ill, and the median age of the homeless chronically ill is significantly lower than before. The universe of a homeless chronic mentally ill person is poorly defined and understood. But an important factor to keep in mind is that it is a diverse group with diverse needs, and it is a fluid, constantly changing population with individuals moving in and out of homelessness and mental illness. Geographic mobility also adds to the difficulty in determining the number of people in this group.

What are the needs of the homeless chronic mentally ill? Again, they are a very diverse group needing a variety of services. Basic needs include: 1) life supports or subsistence needs (housing, food, medical care and psychiatric services, money [income], and jobs); 2) community support programs (screening and referral services, a caring social network, psychosocial rehabilitation services, mental health care, and case management); 3) contact points and mail boxes; and 4) places for bathing and delousing and for keeping and changing clothes.

Which of the above needs is of first priority is an individual matter and varies within the group. One individual may need housing first, another food, another medical care.

As far as housing is concerned, an array of housing options are needed— emergency housing, transitional or temporary housing, permanent housing, and, for some, asylum. Concern was expressed over the lack of housing available, and the limitations this puts on this service system. Although housing may be the most visible need, it is only one of many needs, and provision of housing alone will not solve the problems of the homeless chronic mentally ill.

In the second session, the question was raised of how the homeless chronic mentally ill get that way. For some, it seems to be a matter of default—economic pressures or hardships, or the inability of people who have been marginally able to hold onto homes to continue to do so because of some changing circumstances. Some lose their homes due to mental illness. For some, living in the streets is a more attractive option than using the housing resources currently available. In the past, the hospital would have provided housing for many of these people. Usually this is no longer the case.

There was some discussion of the disadvantages of providing housing by hospitalization and indeed through the mental health system at all. A strong argument was made that there is a negative psychologic factor that results from having all needs met by the mental health system. In doing so, the mental health system forms a trap and isolates the mentally ill from the community. It was suggested that there should be three separate systems to address vocational needs, housing needs, and mental health needs, so that the patient's entire life is not built around the fact that he or she is mentally ill.

What are the barriers to the homeless chronic mentally ill in getting their needs met? Sixteen barriers were identified.

1. Stigma. a) It can be dehumanizing and stigmatizing to enter the mental health system. b) The public stigmatizes the homeless chronic mentally ill and may be reluctant to cooperate in providing services such as housing to them. Thus, to avoid stigma, the homeless chronic mentally ill avoid the mental health care system.
2. Preclusive admission services by which we attempt to treat people who by professional standards do the best and ignore the rest of the population.
3. Intrusiveness. The homeless chronic mentally ill may fear the intrusiveness, loss of control, and loss of freedom that may result from getting involved in the mental health care system.
4. Lack of financial resources that limit what the mental health care system can provide.
5. Catchmenting. The presence of fixed catchment boundaries make it difficult for those with no fixed address or home to receive care.
6. Inappropriate eligibility guidelines which limit access to entitlements such as Supplemental Security Income, food stamps, and so forth.
7. Fragmentation of services.

8. Inappropriate behavioral expectations for a population whose values and aspirations differ from those of the provider.
9. Professional turf issues that lead to conflicts over who provides what services.
10. Lag issues. Time lag that interrupts the continuity of care.
11. Heterogeneity of the population and diversity of treatment needs, and a service system unresponsive to this diversity.
12. Tension with legal barriers and civil rights issues.
13. Lack of an incentive system that provides motivation to patients.
14. Lack of technology to provide adequate care in some cases.
15. Social resistance in that the providers of care live in a very different world than those needing mental health services.
16. The mental illness itself, which may limit the chronic mentally ill person's willingness or ability to seek help.

In the third session, there was a general consensus that homelessness is a significant problem, and questions about governmental policy related to the problems were raised. An argument was made for approaching the problem of homelessness in general without separating out the homeless chronic mentally ill in particular, since this would tend to further segregate them. It was noted that because there are so many homeless, few in government really want to ask about care for them because it would be so expensive to do so. Thus, denial frequently is used to avoid dealing with the problem, or government agencies get involved in the numbers game and minimize the extent of the problem. In the earlier era of more extensive hospitalization, the mental health system supplied housing, but with deinstitutionalization, it ceased to perform this function for most. However, no other agency of government was willing to take responsibility for housing the homeless chronic mentally ill. Now there are conflicts between the federal, state, and local governments as to who should do what, with the result that what needs to be done is not being done, and everyone blames everyone else.

In the earlier sessions, there had been some disagreement about the governmental level at which these problems should be tackled. In the third session, a strong argument was made that initiatives are needed at all levels, but that strong action and mandated control have to exist at the federal level. It was suggested that the federal government needs to identify the homeless chronic mentally ill population and assess needs and provide resources, and that it also needs to study how basic human necessities are provided to the needy in a wage-earning economy. Initiatives must also be undertaken at state and local governmental levels.

It was noted that the care of the homeless should utilize multiple agencies, not just mental health programs. Reference was made to a recent paper coming from the National Association of State Mental Health Program Directors that outlines the comprehensive approach to the homeless. It outlines welfare policies, housing policies, and medical and mental health policies in such a way as to address needs in these diverse areas through different government agencies. In this way all responsibility for care of the homeless chronic mentally ill does not fall on one group.

In conclusion, the homeless chronic mentally ill are a diverse and constantly changing group about whom there are many questions and no simple answers.

Summary Report of Topic IV

What are the obstacles to implementing programs for the chronic mentally ill? What are the financial and control issues in providing services? What are the legal issues associated with providing services for chronic mental illness? What are the problems associated with societal stereotypes of persons with chronic mental illness?

Neal B. Brown, M.P.A., Recorder

It was my pleasure to assist Dr. Joseph Bevilacqua in three separate sessions focusing on this paper. The paper stimulated considerable discussion in each group, and I will attempt to represent the most important issues that were raised by the discussants.

In my position with the National Institute of Mental Health (NIMH) Community Support Program, I can appreciate the emphasis that Dr. Bevilacqua placed on the political dimensions raised by the issues and obstacles in his paper titled *Chronic Mental Illness: A Problem in Politics*. Regardless of their professional training, State Mental Health and State Community Support directors are constantly struggling with the politics of the mental health and social service systems in their quest to improve opportunities and services for individuals with chronic mental illness.

In order to focus the discussion in each session, we divided the issues into four areas that relate to the questions posed to Dr. Bevilacqua. The areas we suggested to the discussants included: 1) issues related to attitudes about professionals and to training, 2) issues related to government and financing, 3) legal issues, and 4) the issues of stigma and stereotyping. There is more information about the first two issues, only because each group had little time to fully discuss the latter two issues.

PROFESSIONAL/TRAINING ISSUES

It is still believed that too many professionals do not relate well to families and continue to blame families for contributing to their family member's illness. (It should be noted that all the participants in the conference took responsibility for their actions and "blaming" was not a factor on any of the conference sessions.)

Much of the discussion on this subject concerned professional training programs. Some people felt that professional teaching models do not adequately reflect new service delivery concepts for the most severely ill. Professional training departments tend not to share what they know about serving the chronic mentally ill. Some questioned whether state mental health agencies have influence over state-supported training programs and whether graduates of such programs have an obligation to work in public mental health programs—both in hospitals and in the community.

There was discussion about the regulations and requirements of many programs that protect the traditional professions. Some people felt that there may be a need for a new profession to care for the chronic mentally ill, while others felt that each profession should find better ways to work with this population. There was some discussion—particularly by consumers—about the growing self-help alternative programs that could affect professional training. There were also some remarks about the extraordinary growth of community college programs that train individuals to work with the chronic mentally ill.

Recommendations

1. In order to increase their knowledge of the changing roles of professionals in community mental health programs, faculty members should be invited to serve on the boards of community programs.
2. State mental health agencies should make special efforts to collaborate with state boards of higher education.
3. The American Psychiatric Association should take the lead on bringing together all the professional disciplines to discuss how to better serve chronic mentally ill people.
4. Services-training-research (STR) model programs should be developed in various regions of the county to promote and disseminate new technologies for the care and treatment of the chronic mentally ill.
5. These STR models should be used to affect professional training programs in order to get new technologies into professional training structures.

6. Community programs should actively recruit student interns.
7. NIMH training programs should be expanded and should emphasize training for serving the chronic mentally ill.
8. Consumers and families should increase their involvement in the development of training curricula in professional schools.
9. A "blue ribbon" panel should be established by the professional groups to review training program curricula and disseminate information in community care for the chronic mentally ill.

GOVERNMENTAL ISSUES

Many people felt that governmental policies and regulations at all levels have not been helpful in developing community-based programs for the chronic mentally ill. Government is often an obstacle to private development of alternative programs, and there has been a lack of coordinated planning between the public and private sectors.

There was discussion about how government funding programs tend to be more directed at filling beds rather than assisting individuals. Questions were raised in each group about moving resources from institutions into the community and developing fiscal incentives for community programs.

Some people were critical of federal funding criteria that only provide reimbursement for medically oriented services for the chronic mentally ill. There was particular concern about the effects of the new diagnostic-related group (DRG) system. Others were critical of the state for deinstitutionalizing to shift the costs to the federal government.

There was agreement that mental health interest, groups, both professionals and advocates, have not always understood government and policies. There was also agreement that the message and directions to government must be clear.

Recommendations

1. Advocates and professionals must affect governmental systems to make sure that decisions are not made by default.
2. Advocates for the chronic mentally ill must be more united.
3. Care of the chronic mentally ill should be considered a societal responsibility.
4. Providers and government officials should collaborate on the implementation of programs.
5. Paid transitional employment for the chronic mentally ill should not be considered part of the trial work period for the client receiving

Supplemental Security Income and Social Security Disability Insurance payments.
6. Medicaid waivers should be promoted for community care of the chronic mentally ill.
7. A voucher system should be investigated for providing money to consumers and families to purchase services.
8. Rehabilitative research and training centers should work with NIMH to develop standards for services to the chronic mentally ill.
9. An alternative model to the DRG system should be offered.
10. There should be more research on service systems issues, that is, moving from hospital to community care.
11. The federal government should look at models and program incentives rather than at program expansion.

LEGAL ISSUES

There was some general discussion about the role of the courts as related to the mental health system. Some people questioned whether the role of the courts should be broadened.

The issue of the chronic mentally ill in the jail system was mentioned in two groups. It was agreed that the mentally ill are not being diverted from jails in most states.

There was considerable discussion about commitment laws in each group. There was some agreement that we were looking at our issue of civil liberties versus family responsibility. There was also agreement that we should separate the issues of confinement from the treatment issues and that decisions in this area will greatly affect the development of community-based care and treatment programs.

Recommendations

1. We should explore program-oriented alternatives to hospital commitment and look carefully at the Wisconsin model.
2. More nonhospital alternatives for people in crisis should be established.
3. We should experiment with psychiatric/community crisis teams to help families.
4. Lawsuits and legislation should be used to define and determine alternatives to hospitalization.
5. A process for coalition to develop a nondivisive response to treatment/ danger issues should be developed.

STIGMA ISSUES

In the brief time available to discuss this area, there was some discussion about stigma among hospital staff, and one person raised a question about whether the mentally ill themselves have added to the stigma problem.

There was agreement that stigma is having its greatest effect on employment of the chronic mentally ill. There were questions about the use of public education approaches for dealing with stigma.

Recommendations

1. Promote the facts about the mentally ill: first, that they are people and are not stupid, and many are certainly courageous.
2. Promote transitional employment programs with special incentives to hire the chronic mentally ill.
3. We should consider suits against some television networks for stigmatizing the mentally ill.
4. We should organize "watchdog groups" over the media.

Summary Report of Topic V

The Role of Families in the Care of the Chronically Mentally Ill: Reactions and Recommendations

R. Don Horner, Ph.D., Recorder

The paper presented by Ms. Shirley Starr reviews the major issues addressed by the 1978 conference on the chronic mental patient (that is, deinstitutionalization, funding of services, training of psychiatrists, service priorities, continuum of community care, housing, employment, and rehabilitation services) as well as some new issues (for example, the growing number of chronic mentally ill persons who are homeless).

The updated information addresses state agency efforts to deflect mentally ill persons from state hospitals, the trend toward subcontracting mental health services to private nonprofit and/or for-profit enterprises, and the declining federal commitment to the mentally ill, as reflected in a diminishing National Institute of Mental Health (NIMH) budget, cuts in research and training funds, and reductions in entitlement programs.

In regard to the role of the nonprofessional, Ms. Starr expressed dissatisfaction with this term and appealed for a different referent. The discussion groups felt that the phrase "friends and family of the mentally ill" was more specific and communicated better about the specific individuals who have valuable roles in regard to mentally ill persons. This led to changing the title of the paper from *Six Years Later: The Role of the Nonprofessional* to *The Role of Families in the Care of the Chronic Mentally Ill*. The groups discussed the roles suggested in the paper and offered many recommendations concerning appropriate roles for friends and family of the mentally ill. These recommendations fell into three major categories: supportive roles, advocacy roles, and monitoring roles.

Supportive Roles

Assistance in locating needed resources. Often both those who actually are experiencing mental illness and family members who want to assist them have limited experience in accessing resources that are available to them. Families can take the initiative and launch a systematic effort to determine what resources are available and what procedures have to be followed to access those resources.

Provide information on mental illness to families or others who know someone experiencing mental health problems. Ignorance is not bliss when the need arises to assist others in caring for someone who experiences a psychotic break, bizarre hallucinations, paranoid delusions, or similar episodes. Having basic information on how to deal with someone demonstrating such behavior as suicidal tendencies can be very important. Having basic information on precursors of mental illness can serve as an early warning system and trigger an offer of assistance. Information on how to assist someone to achieve reintegration into society after an extended hospital stay also can be of great value and may help prevent subsequent return to a hospital environment.

Help those experiencing mental illness develop survival skills. It is well recognized that even those with considerable symptomatology can survive in the mainstream of social life if they have a set of basic living skills. Those who are concerned about the survivability of a particular individual can assist that individual by seeing that the person maintains or acquires the skills that are necessary to meet the demands of everyday life. The behaviors necessary to hold down a job, maintain an acceptable appearance, engage in basic social interaction, and manage one's personal affairs are areas critical to community life. These behaviors can be developed and/or maintained if someone is willing to expend the effort and assist an individual experiencing difficulty in coping with the demands presented by daily life.

Forming networks of mutual support. Many times knowing there is someone who cares, who is available in times of uncertainty or unusual stress, and who can be called upon for support, understanding, and even assistance is sufficient to enable one to cope with situations or events that otherwise might prove unmanageable. Organizing a network of such persons juxtaposed across work, home, leisure, and other components of a person's life space can form a safety net of concern and quick action.

Pulling families into active participation in the treatment of a family member. It is becoming more and more apparent that in many cases one cannot successfully take a family member out of the family context, fix him or her, and return that person ready to cope. The person's family can be a source of conflict or support and sometimes both. If the family becomes an active participant in the treatment of one of its members, the remaining members can learn how to be supportive, how to deal with conflict, and how to make other positive contribution to treatment.

Serving as or developing surrogates for those without active family involvement. The absence of family or friends or anyone who cares about the welfare of an individual can make the course of treatment for that individual an uphill struggle. The availability of someone to serve as a surrogate family member or a concerned friend can be a valuable addition to an individual's life. The offering of emotional support, advice, companionship, and perhaps even financial assistance often can mean the difference between therapeutic success and failure.

Advocacy Roles

Promoting training that will upgrade the skills and knowledge of those involved in such activities as pastoral counseling. There are a number of people who are not direct mental health providers but nevertheless often are called upon to assist those experiencing mental health problems. These individuals, if they have sufficient knowledge and skill, are in a position to be of significant benefit to those experiencing chronic mental illness. Family and friends can advocate that the skills required to make a difference be included in the training programs that prepare individuals to assume such roles as vocational counselor, pastor, general medical practitioner, public health nurse, teacher, and so forth.

Encouraging the offering of incentives to psychiatrists and other mental health professionals to treat those with severe problems of mental health. Many individuals who experience problems of adjustment, stress, anxiety, and so forth often can be helped immediately. This leads some mental health practitioners to focus exclusively on that population. The limits placed on reimbursements, the difficulties in reversing long-standing psychiatric disorders, and the lack of supportive influences such as family, friends, co-workers, and so forth are disincentives to treating those with severe problems of mental health. Incentives such as smaller case loads, greater compensation, and community support systems might be effective in increasing the willingness of psychiatrists and other mental health professionals to offer services to the chronic mentally ill.

Organizing social rehabilitation programs that focus on daily living skills. Many of those with severe problems of mental health have been found to benefit from psychosocial rehabilitation programs. These include social interaction with both those who have experienced problems of mental health and those who have not. Such experiences not only develop important social skills but also help fill the long hours reported by those who do not know what to do with themselves. Advocates have a strong role in serving as organizers of such programs.

Promoting the integration of psychiatry and general medicine. Many families find themselves faced with a member who will not seek any help. In many cases, the only way help can be forced on the member is when problems become so intense that the person is judged to be dangerous to him- or herself or others. Thus, families have to rely heavily on physicians trained in general medicine and its specialties. Advocacy efforts should be directed at increasing the extent to which general medical practitioners are aware of and make effective use of the basic principles of psychiatry.

Proposing systems of service rather than depending on isolated examples of good services here and there. A successful advocacy effort will focus on the broad issues associated with a systemwide need rather than focusing on a specific need in a specific place. The identification of both a pervasive and readily recognized need and an existing mechanism for meeting that need has a better chance of succeeding than isolated attempts to promote services only remotely related to the existing service system.

Threatening and, if needed, taking legal action in those cases in which the basic needs of individuals with problems of mental health are not being met. While legal action is still viewed by many as a means of last resort, others are no longer as content as they once were to wait for change. They wish to force change through the judicial process. Even the threat of a lawsuit still has considerable effect in attracting the attention of those who administer mental health systems. Many of the successful reforms of recent years were the result of suits filed by advocacy groups.

Forming coalitions to deal with issues that require a united front. An example of an issue for which a collective voice might be more effective is the stigmatization of the mentally ill by the media. A coalition of advocacy groups could bring increased pressure to reduce the stereotypic portrayal of individuals with severe problems of mental health. Another concern centers around the need to improve the distribution of information on successful programs. Advocacy groups and organizations should take the initiative to seek and evaluate the results of specific programs and, if found to be successful, advocate for their replication. The evaluation of success may be a particularly meaningful role for families, patients, and ex-patients.

Lobbying for additional funds for research on treatment and prevention of mental illness. It is clear that research is required before both cures and prevention will be forthcoming. Research requires not only the creative capacity of scientific minds but also the funds to enable the experimental verification of proposed solutions. Funds for research are among the most difficult to acquire; thus, skilled lobbying that shows that families recognize the importance of research is crucial if research efforts are to be continued.

Attempting to influence the political process in establishing new and additional services for those experiencing mental illness. This is one of the most traditional (yet continues to be one of the most important) advocacy roles. Most everyone familiar with the political process can attest to the political power of a well-informed and articulate family member pleading the case for new and additional services before a legislative committee. An effective advocacy organization will make certain that its members understand the political and administrative mechanisms that influence services and the specific audience to which recommendations and requests for change must be addressed.

Promoting the establishment of residencies for psychiatrists in community-based programs serving people with long-term mental illness. Most psychiatrists complete residencies in hospital settings. Thus, they do not have a structured opportunity to learn about the types of treatment programs that are successful in less-restrictive settings. Increasing the number of residencies offered through community-based treatment programs eventually should increase the number of psychiatrists who replicate these programs in other settings.

Proposing expansion of community-based services for those with severe problems of mental health. The original concept of community-based services in many states was limited to services that could be provided on an outpatient or consultant basis. This concept has had to be expanded for those with severe mental health problems. The expansion of services to include partial-hospitalization programs, supervised living arrangements, day treatment programs, and so forth is necessary if any agency is to properly serve this group.

Promoting the reduction of the number of individuals with problems of mental health who are also homeless. Advocating the creation of services for individuals who have no place to live is undeniably a high priority. Newspaper and other media accounts of former residents of psychiatric hospitals who are sleeping near steam vents and living in plywood shipping crates, recessed doorways, or abandoned buildings have termed the problem a national disgrace. The problems of establishing shelters, as well as establishing and encouraging use of mental health services for and by shelter residents, are formidable. It will take an intense and consistent advocacy effort to establish services that will result in a significant reduction in the number of mentally ill individuals who are homeless.

Development of guidelines for the placement, treatment, and retention of persons with long-term mental illness in the forensic units of state hospitals and in prisons and development of guidelines for general encounters with the legal system. It is common knowledge that in some states individuals with severe mental illness who commit crimes are committed to the forensic units of state mental health facilities and remain there longer than would have been the case had they been sentenced to prison. While this problem now is receiving more attention than in the past, there is still considerable concern that those with long-term mental illness do not fare well if they happen to encounter the legal system. These individuals need to be represented by advocates who point to these problems and think through appropriate solutions. The families of those who have experienced first hand the inequities suffered by those with mental illnesses are in the best position to articulate the need for reform.

In general, serving as advocates in any area in which professionals may be viewed as having a vested interest. It is not uncommon that members of a survey team who represent a particular discipline find that a facility does not have enough staff to make effective use of that particular professional discipline. Each profession has a vested interest in its particular worth to the mental health field. Rather than entering into rivalries and being caught in the middle between professionals, families should advocate for services that will meet the specific treatment needs of their family member. The advocacy effort also should indicate the types of services that they believe have the most successful influence on the treatment of that member.

Monitoring Roles

Judging the effectiveness of medications in controlling symptoms. Perhaps no one is in a better position to judge the effectiveness of medications in controlling the symptoms of mental illness than close friends and family.

Those who know an individual well and maintain close ties can detect quickly when an individual's medications are excessive, insufficient, and/or ineffective. The offering of information that is rational and well thought out can have a significant impact on a physician or psychiatrist. The presence of any undesirable side effects of certain medications also can be monitored. This could provide quite effective in preventing such disorders as tardive dyskinesia.

Identification of effective programs and communicating this information to those seeking effective programs. Friends and family, through close contact with someone receiving treatment, potentially are in a good position to identify a treatment program as effective, ineffective, or somewhere in between. The positive, neutral, or negative observations, perceptions, and opinions can be provided to others who seek such information. The observations should be clearly labeled as based on limited experience and accompanied by the suggestion that other inquiries be made in an effort to develop as informed a position as possible on the effectiveness of any specific program.

Tracking changes in rules and regulations or legislation that adversely affects those with problems of mental health. This is a very demanding task requiring close and consistent review of publications, laws, and administrative regulations on the national, state, and local levels. Often the rule-making process is not the responsibility of those who have made a systematic effort to address the problem; thus, the problem is not solved by the proposed rule(s). In addition, there often is insufficient experience upon which to judge the potential impact of proposed legislation prior to enactment. For these reasons, tracking proposed and actual changes and predicting or determining from experience their effect on those with problems of mental health is a valuable role for friends and family.

Detecting gaps in the service system that need to be plugged. Friends and family who have been in the position of attempting to locate appropriate services for those experiencing problems of mental health quickly become acutely aware of any gaps in the service system. In addition, they often are a valuable resource in the development of services that can plug these gaps.

Reviewing programs to determine the extent to which they conform to standards of quality accepted as adequate or better. Across the country there are examples of efforts to put friends, family, and other concerned citizens in the role of program reviewer. Mechanisms such as boards of visitors, citizen advisory boards, educational advocates, and so forth are the result of a recognition that citizens can assess quality and provide critical reviews of the extent to which programs adequately conform to recognized standards.

Reviewing television, magazine, newspaper, and other public references to mental illness. It is a common media practice to preface acts of violence and other criminal or bizarre behavior with the referent "a former mental patient" even though such behavior appears no more often in those with problems of mental health than in the general population. Family and friends can watch for such stigmatizing statements and write letters to the editor and ask for equal time to provide a rebuttal, to make the case for avoiding any public declarations that unnecessarily complicate the lives of those with problems of mental health.

The many supportive, advocacy, and monitoring roles were offered by the various discussion groups with varying levels of agreement on the extent to which each was an appropriate role for friends and family of the mentally ill. Each of the above roles had some degree of support, and many received near unanimous support of each discussion group. In general, a consensus evolved that friends and family of the mentally ill are an extremely valuable resource and are likely to become even more valuable as those in close contact with a mentally ill person become more and more a part of that person's treatment process.

Appendix C

National Association of State Mental Health Program Directors Policy Statement on Housing for Chronic Mentally Ill Persons

December 1984

The State Mental Health Directors agree that housing of chronic mentally ill persons is a crucial national problem, one which is integrally involved in successful treatment of this population and which is therefore a very high priority of state mental health authorities.

It is the responsibility of state mental health authorities to take the lead role in addressing this need, advocating for improving the housing situations of these clients and developing specialized residential services for them.

Although public mental health systems need to exercise leadership in this area, addressing these needs is a shared responsibility of mental health authorities, public assistance agencies, public housing authorities, the private sector, and consumers themselves.

An important focus of state mental health activity should be on negotiating mutual roles and responsibilities with local community mental health agencies, as well as the other responsible public and private-sector parties.

Assisting chronic mentally ill persons to improve their housing and provision of intensive residential treatment must take place in the context of an overall community support system. In fact, assistance with housing and residential services should take place concurrently with community support system development, since the number of residential facilities needed may be greatly reduced if adequate vocational, day treatment, and case management services, including assistance in securing and improving housing, are available in a community.

Although historically public mental health systems have provided housing for this population in state institutions, we now recognize that effective treatment principally involves clients living in normal community housing to which mental health authorities provide professionally intensive levels of services.

Financing adequate housing and residential treatment is also a shared responsibility of public housing agencies, public assistance agencies, the private sector, and the public mental health system. Mental health authorities have an important lead role in coordinating the availability of these various funding sources and negotiating in each state the unique mix of financing necessary to meet these needs. In spite of these individual state differences, we agree that:

1. Public mental health systems are responsible for financing or otherwise coordinating the development of the full range of community support services, including assistance to secure improved housing.
2. Public mental health systems are also responsible for directly financing those residential settings that are intensive treatment facilities, rather than housing alternatives per se.
3. Fostering direct provision of housing, or long-term subsidy of housing, is an area in which mental health authorities should also take a lead advocacy role through convening local mental health, public housing, and public assistance authorities, the private sector, consumers, and families to plan a shared approach to improving the housing situations of chronic mentally ill persons.
4. Adequate attention to the housing needs of this group also requires a renewed focus on developing a coordinated federal approach to the respective roles of the Department of Health and Human Services, the Department of Housing and Urban Development, the Veterans Administration, the Health Care Financing Administration, and others in meeting these needs.

National Association of State Mental Health Program Directors Policy Statement on Homelessness for Chronic Mentally Ill Persons

December 1984

Homelessness is a general social problem of increasing magnitude that can be resolved only though the coordinated efforts of governmental welfare, social, health, and mental health programs in conjunction with the private sector. While a minority of homeless people suffer mental health problems, their homelessness is the result of a multiplicity of factors including substance abuse, joblessness, low-cost housing policies, health problems, and so forth. The role of the state mental health authority is to participate in resolving the problem of homelessness by ensuring that the chronic mentally ill are given adequate housing opportunities, either directly or through other governmental agencies, and that all homeless people have access to mental health services.

In addressing the multidimensional problem of homelessness, it is imperative that mental health professionals enter into an immediate, integrated effort with other health and social service providers on federal, state, and local levels to:

- assess the extent and nature of the problem;
- recognize and begin to address the multiplicity of causes of homelessness;
- develop policies, programs, and interventions toward long-term, permanent solutions with the necessary supports to mentally ill homeless persons;
- focus on prevention of homelessness among the mentally ill; and
- initiate a campaign to educate professionals and the public regarding the plight of homeless people, erode the stereotypic images of this population, and decrease public intolerance.

While national as well as local estimates of the number of homeless people are widely divergent, there is a consensus, and it is the position of the National Association of State Mental Health Program Directors (NASMHPD) that the number is significant and steadily growing.

Similarly, there are limited reliable data on the proportion of homeless people also suffering mental disorders. Part of the difficulty in estimating the proportion of homeless people who are mentally ill stems from the fact that conditions such as chronic lack of sleep, poor nutrition, and the stress of life on the street are associated with behavior patterns that may be perceived as manifestations of mental illness. Current estimates are that about 30 percent experience a psychiatric disorder. A sharp increase in the number of young, chronic mentally ill people is also cited in the literature. Part of the problem may be attributable to the changing role of psychiatric inpatient service from custodial to therapeutic without concomitant strengthening of community support systems. This situation, along with other social and economic policies, contributes to homelessness and calls for action by the mental health system. There appear to be a significant number of homeless persons who have a range of mental health problems but have never sought mental health care and are therefore not known to the system. It is the position of NASMHPD that this population must be identified and their needs systematically addressed, both by mental health agencies and through coordination with other related public and private agencies.

A uniform definition of homelessness is essential to any coordinated approach. In this regard, NASMHPD adopts the following definition:

The homeless are defined as people who are without housing on a periodic or permanent basis. The typical plight of homeless persons involves lack of adequate financial resources for basic survival needs such as food and health care.

It is the responsibility of mental health agencies to identify from this population those who are also mentally ill, whether it be as a result of homelessness, causative of homelessness, or coincidence.

The activities listed below represent a range of possible approaches that could be undertaken by mental health agencies to address this complex problem. These activities are not exhaustive and will need to be modified in accordance with regional/local differences.

1. Participate in establishing a coalition of public and private agencies and volunteer and charitable organizations at all levels that will address issues that extend beyond the direct purview of mental health agencies. a) A public policy toward homeless individuals should be established based on the humanitarian principle that the persons, regardless of the cause of homelessness, are entitled to the fulfillment of the basic human needs for shelter and food. It is the obligation of each state to insure that these needs are met. b) Shelter capacity should be expanded to the extent needed to insure that these basic needs are met, but should be viewed as a short-term response to housing problems. c) The number of homeless persons identified in a particular municipality or region should serve as the basis for allocating resources. d) Sufficient resources need to be committed for comprehensive research into the characteristics of the population, causes of homelessness, and special problems of homeless people. e) Volunteer agencies that operate shelters should receive support and consultation particularly with regard to standards, licensure, and linkages to support systems existing in the community. f) An assessment of the current General Assistance and Aid to Families with Dependent Children regulations should be conducted to identify impediments to emergency assistance, such as address requirements; the assessment should also determine whether the level of payment to recipients is adequate. g) Homeless persons should be guaranteed access to clearinghouses for training programs and employment, where appropriate. h) Clearinghouses on a city, county, or state level should be established to coordinate referrals for housing services to locate housing or to organize subsidized home-sharing arrangements. i) States should insure that rental assistance programs for the homeless are developed and that homeless persons have access to these programs. j) Creative financing

programs for the development of rooming houses or boarding and group homes should be initiated to increase the supply of safe and adequate housing for homeless people. k) The number of low-income permanent housing units should be increased through capital funding projects designated for occupancy by homeless persons. l) Local health agencies, particularly those located in urban areas, should expand their activities directed to the homeless population. m) Residential shelters designed to treat populations with special needs such as alcoholics, victims of domestic violence, and families of these persons should be expanded. n) Legislative, administrative, bureaucratic, prejudicial, and other social environmental barriers blocking homeless persons' access to established health and social services should be minimized or eliminated.

2. Identify from the homeless population those who are also mentally ill, or seriously at risk, whether it be a result of homelessness, causative of homelessness, or coincidence.

3. Conduct surveys of community health agencies to identify service gaps in order to provide a basis for the reallocation of resources and staff and to determine the degree to which the agencies are integrated in the planning and implementation of local or county emergency assistance programs.

4. Provide appropriate referral, case follow-up, and outpatient care to mentally ill persons through a continuum of mental health-sponsored supervised and semisupervised residential alternatives.

5. Increase community support services to the young, chronic mentally ill population and other identified at-risk populations.

6. Develop or expand crisis response teams to prevent evictions of mentally ill persons.

7. Develop or expand respite care programs for families or family members with mental illness who are at risk of becoming homeless.

8. Establish multidisciplinary mental health teams that will provide screening, treatment, and case management of the mentally ill at shelters for the homeless and provide outreach and screening at other sites where homeless people are known to congregate.

9. Mental health agencies seeking to provide adequate housing, support, and treatment opportunities need to develop and refine systems that involve homeless persons in the development, evaluation, and implementation of flexible individualized programs.

Appendix D

Additional Comment

This conference recommends, as part of our national, state, and local community support efforts, the development of non-time limited, community-based environments for persons who are experiencing the disabling effects of psychiatric illness and who are not at their best—environments in which the individual's presence is clearly needed and celebrated and within which there are opportunities for truly meaningful involvement and for productive relationships and friendships.

Such programs should serve as a base from which the individual can more effectively utilize medical and psychiatric services, as well as residential, vocational, and educational opportunities available in the community. These programs should place an emphasis on mutual and self-help, provide advocacy for income and medical entitlements and housing, and be actively engaged in reaching out to others who are hospitalized, isolated in the community, or homeless. Such environments should be encouraged to establish both needed housing alternatives and also specially developed relationships with commerce and industry in order to guarantee access to the workplace.

While it is possible that the opportunities provided by such programs exist in the individual's natural world, to the degree that they do not they should be created by the collaboration of mental health workers and persons who have experienced psychiatric illness and need such programs, with support and encouragement from others in the community, including families of the mentally ill.

James R. Schmidt
Executive Director
Fountain House, Inc.

Appendix E

Suggested Additional Reading

Anthony WA, Cohen MR, Cohen BF: The philosophy, treatment process and principles of the psychiatric rehabilitation approach. New Directions in Mental Health 17:67–74, 1983

Bachrach LL: Planning mental health services for chronic patients. Hosp Community Psychiatry 30:387–393, 1979

Bachrach LL: Overview: model programs for chronic mental patients. Am J Psychiatry 137:1023–1031, 1980

Bachrach LL: Young adult chronic patients: an analytical review of the literature. Hosp Community Psychiatry 33:189–197, 1982

Bachrach LL: An overview of deinstitutionalization, in Deinstitutionalization. Edited by Bachrach LL. New Directions for Mental Health Services, no. 18. San Francisco, Jossey-Bass, 1983

Bachrach LL: The Homeless Mentally Ill and Mental Health Services: An Analytical Review of the Literature on the Homeless Mentally Ill. A Task Force Report of the American Psychiatric Association. Edited by Lamb HR. Washington, DC, American Psychiatric Association, 1984

Cutler DL, Bloom JD, Shore JH: Training psychiatrists to work with community support systems for chronic mentally ill persons. Am J Psychiatry 138:98–101, 1981

Falloon IRH, McGill C, Boyd J: Behavorial Family Management. Baltimore, Johns Hopkins University Press, 1984

Goldstein MJ (ed): New Developments and Intervention with Families of Schizophrenics, New Directions for Mental Health Services, no. 12. San Francisco, Jossey-Bass, 1981

King LW, Kuehnel TG (eds): The Chronic Patient: Treatment and Rehabilitation. Los Angeles, Rehabilitation Research and Training Center, University of California, Los Angeles, 1983

Knitzer J: Unclaimed Children: The Failure of Public Responsibility to Children and Adolescents in Need of Mental Health Services. Washington, DC, Children's Defense Fund, 1982

Lamb HR: Treating the Long Term Mentally Ill: Beyond Institutionalization. San Francisco, Jossey-Bass, 1982

Leepson M: The homeless: growing national problem. Washington, DC, Congressional Quarterly, 29 October 1982

Liberman RP, Foy DW: Psychiatric rehabilitation for chronic mental patients. Psychiatric Annals 13:539–545, 1983

Liberman RP, Kuehnel TG, Phipps CC, et al: Resource Book for Psychiatric Rehabilitation: Elements of Services for the Mentally Ill. Los Angeles, Rehabilitation Research and Training Center, University of California, Los Angeles, 1985

Pepper D, Ryglewicz H (eds): The Young Adult Chronic Patient. New Directions for Mental Health Services, no. 14. San Franscisco, Jossey-Bass, 1982

Talbott JA: Public policy on chronically mentally ill. Am J Orthopsychiatry 50:43–53, 1980

Talbott JA (ed): The Chronic Mentally Ill: Treatment, Programs, Systems. New York, Human Science Press, 1981

Talbott JA (ed): The Chronic Mental Patient: Five Years Later. Orlando, FL, Grune and Stratton, 1984

Woy JR, Goldstrom KD, Manderscheid RW: The Young Chronic Mental Patient: Report of a National Survey. NIMH publication no. OP79-0031. Rockville, MD, National Institute of Mental Health, 1982